MY LIFE IS A PUZZLE

First Published in 2024 by Echo Books

Echo Books is an imprint of Superscript Publishing Pty Ltd
ABN 76 644 812 395

Registered Office: PO Box 669, Woodend, Victoria, 3442

www.echobooks.com.au

Copyright © Rebecca Sharrock

National Library of Australia Cataloguing-in-Publication entry.

Creator: Rebecca Sharrock, author.

Title: My Life Is A Puzzle

ISBN: 978-1-922603-65-4 (paperback)

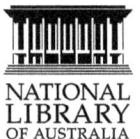 A catalogue record for this book is available from the National Library of Australia

Design by Andrew Davies.
Cover image: Rebecca Sharrock

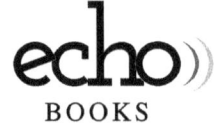

MY LIFE IS A PUZZLE

Rebecca (Catherine) Sharrock

Contents

Introduction	My Memory Condition and Writing Career	7
Section One	**Early Years**	13
One	Welcome to the World Rebecca	14
Two	Who's Who and What's That?	24
Three	Life is Not the Same for Me Anymore	30
Four	Adjusting to Life Within a Family of Three People	35
Five	I'm Now Feeling Ready to Grow Up	41
Six	A New House to Always Call Home	46
Section Two	**Struggles with Autism**	53
Seven	School is not as Great as I Thought it Would Be	54
Eight	I'm a Happy Child but I Do Have Certain Fears and Phobias	60
Nine	Forming Friendships with Peers from Mutual Interests	65
Ten	Nighttime Terrors	68
Eleven	My First Experience of Travelling Overseas	73
Twelve	Now I Actually Want to Spend More Time with My Friends than Doing my Schoolwork	79
Thirteen	My Life is Changing Whether I Want it to or Not	81
Fourteen	Adjusting to a New School with New Friendships to Make	85

Section Three	**More Family and Diagnoses**	93
Fifteen	A Depressing Time with Positive Distractions	94
Sixteen	It's Now Known That I Have Autism	100
Seventeen	Where do I Go to from Here?	108
Eighteen	Traveling Forward into New Beginnings	117
Nineteen	Now I Have to Create My Own Life Path	124
Twenty	Receiving an Unexpected Inheritance and my Black Belt	128
Twenty-One	My Final Year of Uncertainty	133

Section Four	**A New Day Dawns**	137
Twenty-Two	Welcome to the Next Phase of Life	138
Twenty-Three	Navigating the World of Social Media	152
Twenty-Four	Getting Diagnosed with Highly Superior Autobiographical Memory	160
Twenty-Five	Unexpected Surprises	165
Twenty-Six	Little Do I Know How Much My Life Will Change	177
Twenty-Seven	Losing Two Grandfathers for Very Different Reasons	182
Twenty-Eight	Doing Constant Media Interviews is a Full Time Job	210
Twenty-Nine	Accepting that I'm Not Quite Ready for Full Independence	219
Thirty	Coming to Terms with the Reality of Life	268

MY MEMORY CONDITION AND WRITING CAREER

My name is Rebecca (Catherine) Sharrock, and since the very beginning of my life I have had an unusual inability to forget, and emotionally let go of the vast majority of my past experiences. Throughout my childhood and teenage years neither I, my family, nor any medical experts understood why this was the case. It was a complete mystery to us all until 2011, when I was 21 years old. That was when we discovered from a *60 Minutes* episode that a very rare memory condition exists, which is called HSAM (or Highly Superior Autobiographical Memory).

This particular condition was officially discovered by neuropsychologists in 2006, and it makes a person unable to forget the vast majority of their life experiences. Additionally, it also causes one to emotionally relive their past via flashbacks. These flashbacks are both constant and involuntary.

Since birth I had been living my life that way, and previously it had been speculated as being a symptom of another condition I have, which is Obsessive Compulsive Disorder (OCD). However, in contrast to what is typically associated with OCD, the memories I would constantly relive weren't solely from past experiences that had any personal significance. In fact most of those memories were just from very mundane experiences, or 'useless pieces of clutter' as I like to call them.

Of course, I had no knowledge of calendars, months, or even age in my earliest part of life. Yet all of my memories are in chronological order and I remember every single birthday I have ever had. Of course, I didn't fully understand what a birthday was until I turned five. Though I did understand that I didn't get gifts, birthday cards, greetings of 'Happy Birthday', a cake and candles to blow out on every day of the year.

In my earliest years, prior to beginning primary school I would constantly ask my mother questions about meals we ate many months beforehand, and everything in regards to what we did in the past. This was from the moment when I could form simple sentences, (roughly) at the age of around two and a half years old.

Over and over again as a toddler I would hear the phrase "I don't know Becky, it was a long time ago". However, there was a moment when I was sat on my bed at the age of three, and I said "But, one day right now *will* be a long time ago". My mother's reply with a smile was "Yes, and when that time comes you won't remember it". That past experience has now become a very amusing topic of conversation!

This unusual characteristic tends to occur in the lives of people with HSAM; and once we first heard about the condition existing, both I and my family members immediately associated this with my own life.

My parents were regular viewers of the television show *60 Minutes*. The moment they saw an episode featuring the topic of HSAM, was when they finally uncovered the answer to all of our previous questions. They recorded that episode and showed it to me a few days afterward (on Sunday, January the 23rd, 2011).

As I was watching it, I couldn't understand why the recollections of the people featured were considered to be so unusual. After I had queried my parents about this, my mother then expressed how she believed that I myself had this condition. Mum also asked me if I felt okay about her sending the researchers (who discovered HSAM) an email. I accepted, however I knew that we would be one of many millions of people calling in, so I wasn't at all expecting any kind of reply.

Amazingly though, we did receive a reply a mere couple of weeks later, and the researchers said that they were willing to give me their tests!

Then two years later, after numerous kinds of assessments conducted by the McGaugh/Stark Lab at the UCI (University of California, Irvine), I was diagnosed by them as having HSAM in 2013. These tests were done via Skype, email and Zoom. There was also an MRI done of my brain, which involved me having to travel over to California in person.

Then, in May of 2016 the University of Queensland (UQ) began an additional study of my HSAM. It's very interesting how the researchers and neuropsychologists from each team have their own individual areas of focus.

Also, in the early days a large number of people who would hear of me participating in all of this HSAM research would query me, in regards to what the exact purpose of it was, for both science and myself.

In answer to this, I always say that in addition to gathering self-knowledge about my kind of memory and psychology, being involved in HSAM research tests gives me something to work on. Especially in my early adulthood, it was essential for me to gradually develop the skills I needed for a job. Previously I hadn't been given such a potentially effective opportunity to do so.

It's true that I'll never live a life that many would consider to be 100% independent. Yet to have now risen to a score of being around 75% independent (in comparison to being around 15% independent shortly after leaving school) this is something that my family, doctors and even myself are very satisfied with. Despite not being quite to the same level as most of my same age peers, a decade ago none of us ever expected my life skills to be where they are today.

All of my family and friends are equally satisfied with this whole independence journey (from birth to 30 years old). That complex journey has also been included in the following chapters that you're about to read! As well, after reading this whole book you will discover the exact meaning of all of the four dates that I printed on the glass cube of its cover page. This book about my life truly is a puzzle for the reader to solve!

Shortly after learning how to speak in words, I became very interested in learning another primary form of communication, which is to read and write. Once I had learned how to read children's Disney books and encyclopaedias, I was very interested in creating my own written material. This I now do by writing books and blogs.

My enjoyment of practicing writing has continued to the present day, which is the main reason for why I decided that writing books would be a great hobby for me. Yet, I always knew that there were a few very significant obstacles that I would have to work through before I could both write and get a book published.

Despite how much I have always enjoyed writing, I am very limited when it comes to understanding emotions, as well as creating new ideas and stories by using imagination. Many are very surprised to hear me say this because I have loved to write, draw and build things with toy bricks since my early childhood. However just about everything that I create has to be based upon a model that already exists. Thus I have almost always drawn and painted still-life pictures (both from photos and from personal memories). As well, all of the things that I create with Lego and on Minecraft are from structures, scenery and towns that already exist. My guides for those creations come from photos, film, Google Earth or from memory.

In regards to written work, it's a very similar story. I do much better with writing non-fiction in comparison to creative fiction. Also, I only write nonfiction pieces in either a first person or a third person format. Despite my material still being original, it has to be based on given fact, or on personal experiences that I remember happening to me. This is so much so that even writing hypotheses and 'up in the air' theories creates much mental struggle.

So, in other words I still absolutely love writing material, just as long as it's done in my own individual way. The style of writing that is ideal for me is to document facts or personal memories in chronological order, from x to x. Ideally that would be more suitable for writing an autobiography of everything significant that has happened from my earliest days to the present time.

Though a short phase of my life came which caused me to put my goal of writing a book to the back of my mind, temporarily. From the years 2011 to 2013 I was very busy with all of the diagnostic tests given to me by neuropsychologists at the University of California, Irvine (UCI).

Not too long ago, I was so preoccupied with finding a reason for why I constantly relive both happy and painful memories, that I previously had no time to even consider working on a book.

Though, as soon as I began to be featured in media stories, a large number of people asked me if there was a book available, which included more details about all the life experiences that I've mentioned in my interviews.

The answer was of course no, *but* my old passion (that had been buried amongst other things that got in the way) was rekindled. I did after all always have a desire to write a book, which would be a chronological memoir about all of my significant life experiences.

It would obviously be impossible to write down events from literally every second of my life in a book! That would take more than three decades!

So for the past three years I've been writing up (relevant) material for this book, *My Life is a Puzzle*. It's name has come from the visualisation I get whenever I'm sorting through my life, memories and emotions. While I was writing down all of my significant life experiences into this book, I was indeed working on this puzzle of my life. My life truly *does* feel exactly like working on a jigsaw or Rubik's cube whenever I try to make sense of it all.

Also, in August of 2022 a film about myself and my family (unique in the sense that we ourselves play our own roles) will be premiered at the Melbourne International Film Festival. My intention is to release my book around the same time as our movie, which has been named *Because We Have Each Other*.

Whenever comments have appeared on media sites of whom I do interviews with, the vast majority that I see are so kind and uplifting.

I've also developed such a wonderful group of friends worldwide who like myself have autism, Obsessive Compulsive Disorder or HSAM.

Lastly, it's very important for me to mention that I am not the only person diagnosed with each of the conditions that I have. So this book is not a representation of every case of autism, Obsessive Compulsive Disorder or HSAM. It merely follows the life journey of one person who just happens to have those three conditions.

SECTION ONE

EARLY YEARS

CHAPTER ONE

WELCOME TO THE WORLD REBECCA

I was born in Brisbane, Australia on December the 11th, 1989 (at 6:55am to be precise) and my recollections go back to somewhere around that time. Yet those memories can not of course be confirmed with a date. The way my recall works is that I remember events in a chronological sequence. So whenever a very early memory has a confirmed date attached, I'll have a rough idea of what happened to me a few days before or afterward. As a newborn, I had no awareness of what calendar dates were, and they can of course only be confirmed by photos and other people's recollections.

This means that despite how much I know and feel emotionally that those extremely early recollections are truly memories, there is no possible way of giving 100% proof to a skeptic, if I were recalling an experience from when I was too young to know about calendar dates. Also, whenever I have come across people who are skeptical about my HSAM, I don't feel anger or aggression towards them.

Even though some have said things to me that are especially hurtful, I still understand that they can only believe what they can see for themselves. It's not possible for me to give an accurate account of what I personally see and feel by solely using words (even if I were more verbally articulate).

As well, I've learned in recent years that there *are* people in the world who are low enough to lie about having rare medical conditions, simply and appallingly for the purpose of receiving attention. They also mistakingly believe that they will get immense fame and fortune by doing so.

In truth having HSAM is very challenging and I require weekly therapy as a result of it, in order for me to be able to live a healthy life. As human beings we're not biologically supposed to have this inability to let go of the past, and having an extremely rare condition is very difficult because there are not many resources available to help us with it. Additionally, being one of few people with a certain condition can often make us feel very lonely, and even medically disregarded at times.

There's also very little that autobiographical recall can be used for in a career, so it's definitely a myth that HSAM makes you exceptionally wealthy. Contrary to many of the beliefs of people I come across, having your story published in all kinds of media shows/news articles is voluntary work. So there would be absolutely no purpose for anyone to make the whole story up, and it would therefore be completely worthless to dig such a deep hole for myself from such a pointless lie.

As mentioned previously it is very difficult for me to prove my earliest recollections to skeptics, mainly because of today's general assumption of it being impossible for people to remember prior to a certain age; and additionally from a person being unable to date their earliest experiences due to being so young at the time.

Though in a relatively recent interview I was asked to cast my mind back as far as it could possibly go. My first response was that I'd be unable to give a fully confirmed date. All I could give was a rough estimate based on the amount of time before and after other experiences, which *were* dated.

However during this particular interview I was asked to just put those things aside, and voice my earliest memory regardless. So here we go...

When I stretch my mind back to the very beginning of my existence (as a person developed enough to have a sense of self) I recall being enclosed with my head tucked in between my legs. At that time I hadn't known life any differently so I had no discomfort from being trapped in such a small place. I did not think much of my surroundings, as there really wasn't anything interesting to think about. Perhaps too, I wasn't yet developed enough to have sophisticated thoughts and feelings. It was the only environment I had ever seen and felt, and I had long since learned all I needed to know about it.

This is assumed by many (including myself) as being from when I was a well developed foetus in the womb. However this memory could very well have been from when I was wrapped in a blanket just after I was born. As I said before, the details I can solely give of this past experience aren't nearly enough for a skeptic to consider as being legitimate.

Even though I strongly believe it's from when I was in the womb, other people can rightfully argue against this because there is little proof.

Also, I don't have any recollections of being two reproductive cells in different bodies (those of my mother and father), and there are not many recollections of me being in an assumably womb-like environment covering the whole length of nine months.

Another early recollection is of me being laid down and having something clipped to my ankle. This happened at a chronologically later stage from that previous memory of me being scrunched up in a foetal position, and it was prior to my first (dated) memory. If I had felt something being clipped to my ankle, this was most likely from the moment just after my birth.

Interestingly as a newborn I hadn't yet developed the urge to go forward and physically explore what such curious objects could be, despite having a huge amount of curiosity about the world in which we live. At that age I was indeed very curious, yet not in an explorative and expansive kind of way. In other words I merely felt curious about the *physical* details of everything around me, and hadn't yet reached the stage where I questioned *why* everything existed the way in which it did. As well, prior to knowing any language I did not think and reason in words. Instead I did so purely by emotions and information given to me through my five senses. It was so much quicker to think that way, and regardless of how much I've been attempting to, I can not retrain myself to do so again in the current day.

Many a time I've been asked about whether or not it felt strange that I'd been in my mother's womb (and had not yet been born) a mere week or so beforehand. My answer is always that I lived purely in the *present* moment at that age.

So as a newborn, it felt no different to think of myself not existing a year earlier then, than it does from when I think of not yet existing forty years earlier than today. Nowadays I've lived the length of a year many times before, and I now know it to not be a long time. Yet at the stage when I was a newborn, I had never known anything as long as a year before. So a year sounded like an enormous amount of time. Perhaps the reason for why life seems to increasingly pass by more quickly as we age is because we become more familiar with larger stretches of time.

Also, at that age I didn't ever think about the concept of there being a past, present and future. All I acknowledged was living in the moment. Despite having had memories much in the same way as I do now (in a chronological sequence), the concept of there being a 'past' wasn't something I had yet fully understood consciously.

Deep down I did know there was a past. Yet at an extremely young age it was too complex a concept for me to even give acknowledgement to. Birth, growing up, ageing and death were all subjects that I didn't understand, and nor did I give any thought to them at the time.

During my very early ages I had no knowledge of calendars, dates, days or numbers (nor the names of them). Despite not knowing the definition of what a day was at that time, I did still recall the cycles of day and night which I had experienced. Thus from the knowledge I have today I can roughly figure out how many days (or perhaps even months) occurred before or after an early event that I now have a confirmed date for. This could be from either a photograph or an event like my birthday or Christmas Day.

The earliest memory (that I can date) is from when I was twelve days old. Mum was carrying me in a cotton blanket to the front seat of the car, which was my father's idea. By that time I was already familiar with being held, and I always knew when it was my mother who was holding me. This wasn't just by sight either. It was mainly by instinct. My guess for this, as a very amateur psychologist, is that I had a subconscious understanding of my mother's feel and temperament, due to having previously lived within her for almost a year.

I was then gently placed down on the car seat and had a picture taken of me looking up at the steering wheel. In addition to the steering wheel, the camera also grabbed my attention.

Cameras of that day were much bigger than those of today's time. Therefore they were just about impossible to miss for a sighted person, even for a short-sighted person when they're not wearing artificial lenses (as has been the case for me since I was twelve *years* old). Though after a few months, I definitely got used to having my picture taken. Many parents just cannot help taking constant pictures of their children! I can't even imagine how it would feel now for a baby born in the current age of social media, where everyone has such easy access to mobile devices with cameras, and pictures taken can be shared instantly!

I would discuss this 'twelve days old' recollection many times with my mother, and for quite some time it remained to be one of those very early yet unconfirmed past experiences that I have.

However there was one afternoon at the age of thirteen (years) when I was looking through some old family photos. These included those of my parents, grandparents, myself and my biological sister Jessica. As I was flicking through them, a moment came when I paused on a particular photograph (which very sadly has now become lost in the sands of time) that I had in my hand.

It was dated 23/12/1989 and I saw a picture of a newborn child laying down on a car seat. The baby was also on a sheepskin carseat cover, which was the exact surface I remembered myself having been laid down onto many years beforehand. After seeing other parts of my previous surroundings, I quickly realised that this was a picture of the experience I would constantly tell my mother about, and I rushed to show her the picture!

When mum saw both the photograph and the date on it, she was puzzled as to how I could remember an experience from when I was so young. In 2003 (when I was thirteen years old for most of the year) we had no idea that I had HSAM or even about what the condition was.

So despite how much she publicly boasts of me having remembered this now, mum was initially rather skeptical back in the year 2003! She was asking me about how I could possibly remember an experience from when I was less than a fortnight old. Though after emphatically insisting with passion that I did truly recall that experience, and from adding in other details which weren't photographed, (including the appearance of all the people present at our house on that day), mum was finally convinced after roughly half an hour of listening to me!

Returning to the very act of learning how to talk in the first place, it was something that developed at a gradual pace, and that began from the very moment I was born (or within a week of my birth). It didn't take me long to instinctively figure out that people around me were making sounds to communicate, despite not understanding a word of what they were saying at first.

At the very beginning of my life I had not yet learned a first language. So it was much harder than learning French and Spanish is for me today, as I now have English words and sentence structure as a guide. Even if words are enormously different, I now have references such as "Perro means dog in Spanish", or "Fromage means cheese in French". Also, as a newborn I additionally had many limitations with my cognitive skills.

Despite having a much stronger ability with absorbing new information at that previous time, all of the other cognitive skills that I had were frustratingly limited. Of course, I hadn't ever known myself to have greater abilities than what I had back then. But given that I had 1000% more curiosity than I do today, as well as such an intense thirst to learn new skills, I did feel a lot of impatience when I purely and simply couldn't do the vast majority of things that I saw adults around me doing.

Today as an adult myself, my vocabulary has increased a lot more, and I can now give a name (such as impatience and frustration) to that previous feeling. Also, unlike then I can now express my feelings in words.

Initially I realised that crying brought my mother (as well as other people) to me. So it wasn't difficult for me to come to the conclusion of using tears and bawling as a method of somehow communicating prior to language. Yet we all know that babies cry a lot more than adults/ older children, in both frequency and volume! Therefore, skeptical people are perfectly correct when they say that a person doesn't need to remember their infancy to know this.

But whenever I needed assistance or company I would cry. It's true that back then I knew how to manipulate people! But to be fair, it was the only method of communicating that I at first had the ability to use.

As a very young child, another major difficulty for me was that I didn't yet have the cognitive ability to form an organised group of sounds (in the right sequence) as we have to do whilst speaking in any language. However this didn't stop me from trying! For quite some time (almost from the moment when I was born) I would practice making vocal sounds. This may have come across as mere babbling, but in truth I was doing this for the hope of one day being able to talk. Infancy is in most ways a very simple stage of our life, so there doesn't appear to be a lot of personality and cognitive aspects of ourselves to read too far into. However our earliest months and years also appear to be the most interesting, purely because we perceive the world and generally think in a different way to how we do so in our adult life.

Due to the early cognitive difficulties mentioned above, I didn't have the ability to form many words, let alone sentences during my first year. Initially I began speaking by mostly saying single words with one syllable (even words repeating the same syllable like 'ma-ma'). Gradually my skills built up in order for me to start speaking more fluently.

In fact this process didn't stop once I became a toddler, older child or even a teenager. My ability to communicate is continuing to develop to this very day from me adding new words to my vocabulary, as well as from me learning foreign languages in addition to English.

Another skill of which no person is born knowing how to do (successfully at the very least) is the action of walking. Most of us begin taking our first successful steps in our very early toddler years. Prior to that time we require other means of getting around. For some people (including some friends and family of mine with a physical disability) this is lifelong.

So just as is the case with developing speech and other kinds of skills, not every person reaches milestones at the same age. In my own case I began walking and speaking at the typical milestone age, but there were other skills that took me much longer than usual to develop.

When it came to walking, there was a brief stage of my life when I was unable to do so. At first I much preferred to be carried rather than being put into a stroller. Being held was more emotionally comfortable for me, and it felt far less impersonal. Up until the age of approximately six months, my mother would carry me around, either in her arms or in a capsule.

Though at that early stage of my life I didn't yet understand the concept of a child growing with the passage of time. If I were to place my current adult brain into the mind of myself back then, I would easily know that I had grown. This would have been from the shrinking size surrounding me in my crib, the hundred or so clothes I had outgrown, the people around me becoming slightly smaller (in my eyes), as well as the fact that I was gradually getting less room in my capsule.

The strangest part in regards to me talking or thinking about those much earlier recollections nowadays, is that I'm having to put the mind and understanding of such a young child into my current adult mindset. There are so many examples (including that of which I previously mentioned) of facts and answers being right in front of my eyes; though it was only when I looked over memories of those experiences at an older age when I could finally acknowledge those very conspicuous things.

What is even more puzzling for me is that these personal recollections aren't hypothetical scenarios, or another person's words that I'm hearing. It's a very strange feeling when I struggle to understand a mindset that I *myself* previously had, and that I don't have now. How on earth could I possibly not notice myself outgrowing clothes and physical space?! It's mind-boggling!

Though a time came when I finally became too big for my mother to carry me around all the time. The final day of me being carried in my original blanket was when mum went out shopping, some time in between birth and first birthday (I was also a tall baby and child). So my guess is that I was about nine months old.

Despite being unable to reason to the same level that I do now, I was still able to understand regular routines and activities. Thus at the approximate age of nine months I received a surprise when I made a routine movement towards my blanket, and my mother didn't accept the action. I remember her saying "No, you're too big for that now". Those words were not immediately understood by me, so I had to hear that phrase repeatedly before the new procedure of being pushed in a stroller became routine.

For the next year and a half I had to be in a stroller during outings, which I didn't favour too much, and as soon as I could successfully walk I didn't want to go in it at all. To this very day I don't like looking at strollers and I despise the look of the canopies on them. As a baby I absolutely hated having a canopy over my head (however there are other babies who do like them). My mother understood this, so she never had my head covered whilst I was in a stroller.

Shortly before my first birthday I learned how to walk. Learning how to walk was quite a different experience from learning how to talk. I had noticed people both walking and talking since I very first entered this world. As mentioned a little earlier, I quickly realised that people around me were communicating in some way, and I almost instantly began practicing vocal noises to try and develop the ability myself. However it was a little while before I developed an interest in learning the skill of walking. Perhaps it was because so much of my time and energy was spent in learning other things like talking, communicating and mentally exploring the world around me.

But I finally reached a stage when I desired to learn how to walk myself. By then I had learned that crawling enabled me to move around, and by instinct I knew that walking also enabled me to move closer to things (of course this wasn't rationalised in words). I'm not completely sure as to why I quickly and suddenly became interested in the action of walking at a certain time, despite having seen people around me doing so for a year. Though I guess that's just another one of life's many mysteries.

There was one day shortly before my first birthday when I was on the living room floor and my mother was gesturing for me to crawl towards her. Perhaps it had something to do with my autism, but crawling was never an action that I took a liking to. The way I moved felt so uncoordinated, and I felt so awkward whenever I crawled. I much preferred to shuffle. Yet after seeing my mother continuing to gesture for me to do so for several minutes, I clearly realised that she wanted me to move to the other side of the room.

On that day I was determined not to crawl, however to make the experience more interesting I instead stood up and attempted to move towards my mother on two legs. Instinctively I knew the action of putting one foot before the other. Though initially it felt very awkward, even more so than crawling did, and I fell over countless times. For a split second I considered just giving up and remaining on the ground. But instead of simply giving up I more rather felt even more determined to get it right. So I'd get up again, and would walk as fast as I could before I fell over. Eventually there came a time when I was no longer falling at all, and walking then became a luxury that I took for granted.

As I progressed through the next year of my life (and beyond) the number of things that I learned, only to give very little thought to afterward, grew increasingly larger.

CHAPTER TWO

WHO'S WHO AND WHAT'S THAT?

Despite not having any clear recollections from the day I was born (even though there are some very early recollections which *could* be from the day when I was born), I do remember each birthday I had after then. It is true that I didn't understand what my birthday was until I was five years old. However I did indeed know that the day was special because I got showered with so much attention and toys.

On my first birthday I realised that the day was different when my mother was putting me in a nice though very itchy satin dress. I was crying because it was so unlike my usual clothes, primarily made of cotton. Though my mum was explaining to me that it was my very own day, and that lots of people were coming to see me. I heard all of this, and only understood around half of the words she was saying to me, at that time. Yet I was unable to tell my mother that the dress was uncomfortable, or to ask her about the reason for why that day was so special. All I could do was cry, but I did stop less than an hour later when I became distracted by everything else.

By the end of that day I felt reasonably happy. I was given a cake where I had to blow out a curious substance (a flame) on top of a candle, even though I got a nasty shock when I touched the flame and it burnt my finger! With that I screamed briefly out of pain.

Mum wasn't there when it happened and the person supervising me relit the candle by the time she came back. This person also didn't stop or warn me in any way, as my hand reached out towards the flame. So she didn't know what happened until many years later, and was upset that I was unable to tell her at that earlier time.

For that birthday I was given a Minnie Mouse plush toy by my parents, but I was absolutely terrified of it. I would cry every time it was shown to me because I found her wide smile and bright colours to be very scary. I wasn't able to tell my parents that the toy frightened me back then. All I could do at that time was cry and toss it away. However I told my mum about this when I was several years older, and it has become an amusing topic to discuss ever since. I can almost say that the face of Minnie Mouse looked nightmarish to me back then. Yet soon would come the time when I began having actual nightmares.

At the age of about one and a half (not long before my second birthday) I began to dream whenever I fell asleep. Prior to that time I never had dreams. But once I started to dream it made going to sleep an unsettling experience for me. As a one year old I didn't understand that my own mind created dreams. At that time I believed that I really was being taken away from my home.

There was one night when I had gone to sleep as usual, and I had suddenly found myself in a room which was much like a playroom or a jungle gym. Yet instead of being filled with foam balls, it was full of every kind of fruit! Amongst all of the chaos and noise, I spotted a ball and chute machine. It caught my interest because there were countless oranges rolling down the chute and then falling into a box underneath. However the moment I went to the box to search for the stickers on the oranges, I found myself fully awake in my dark bedroom.

The sensation was very frightening and I hoped that I would never experience this again. Yet I was wrong. Night after night I would repeatedly have those 'ventures'. Also, as has always been the case, whenever I was dreaming I was aware that I was doing so, and I would try with all my might to wake up.

So as a result of that I would do everything I could to prevent myself from falling asleep in the first place. I tried holding my eyelids open and would scream, in the hope that it would keep me awake. As well, waking up in the middle of the night after having a dream was additionally unsettling, because it felt dark and lonely and I knew that I would have to again fall asleep. So I'd scream as loud as I could in the hope that my mother would come to me. Her presence would remind me that I hadn't been taken away anywhere, and that I was indeed still at home.

Screaming did bring my mother to me, though as a one year old I didn't have any consideration as to how difficult that would be for my parents. However Mum heard from a friend that tying a large rag doll to a child's crib had proven itself to be useful. This did indeed work (for me) because when it was dark the doll looked much the same as my mother.

I would also see this doll during the day. Though surprisingly I was unable to grasp the fact that it was the exact same comforting figure who stood over me in the dark every night.

As I was leaving babyhood and entering early childhood, there was something else which was giving me a fair deal of anxiety. Inwardly I didn't feel comfortable about socialising with other children and adults. This continues to the present day, and it hasn't got anything to do with me disliking other people. It's merely due to communication and understanding/reading emotions not being an easy thing for me to do.

Whenever I'm struggling to communicate I also experience additional fears of being pressured and judged. This doesn't necessarily mean that I am a shy person, because I never feel that I lack confidence in social settings! Indeed I feel that I can be too self-expressive on many occasions! But it does mean that I feel a lot of pressure when I'm living in a world where constant verbal communication and an instinctive understanding of facial expressions/body language are not only accepted, but expected.

Many a time I say (and truly do believe) that the language of emotion is the hardest language for a person to learn. The part which I find particularly difficult is when I have to understand another person's emotions, because I cannot see and experience them myself. Understanding my own emotions is much easier because I am personally experiencing them with each of my senses and thoughts. It's not at all a result of me having a lack of interest in other people's lives, as several have believed.

Alas, in my day to day life I have always felt much frustration. This was an even more difficult situation in the first couple of decades of my life.

Nowadays I'm still experiencing those feelings, but I recognise them within myself and know that I must control them. Though as a child (and even as a teenager and younger adult) I hadn't yet developed any sort of coping mechanism for those feelings I experience today. So there were many daily meltdowns, to various intensities for a *very* long time.

When I was a young toddler my mother thought it was a good idea for me to begin doing outings at a local playgroup. This was for the purpose of developing my social skills for preschool and school later on. Mum would also be there with me. At the time it was not yet known that I had autism or any anxiety disorders. Despite having exactly the same characteristics back then as I do now as an adult, it's very difficult for other people to notice those specific differences in such a young child. After all, one year olds don't typically interact with other people very well, they are very self centred, and their expected inability to handle emotions as effectively as an adult (or as an older child) often masks anxiety disorders too.

While I was at the local playgroup one day, there was a moment when I was given a packet of salt and vinegar crisps while I was sitting on the swing. I could smell the bark beneath me and I was entertained by examining my packet of crisps. Mum had opened the packet for me and I was fascinated by that action, which back then I had no idea of how to do myself. The open end of this packet was of great interest to me, and it wasn't long before I became interested in the closed end. As I was comparing the open and closed side I turned the packet upside down. Unfortunately all of my crisps fell on to the floor, which I was unable to predict happening. Mum then said that they were all gone, and I burst into tears! However that wasn't the final time when I made a similar error.

Not long after then, my parents and I went on a family trip down to Mansfield, in Victoria. My parents decided to drive down there instead of taking a flight. So it was a very long car trip from our home in the Brisbane suburb of Paddington. During the road trip I couldn't comprehend what I saw us drive past. Indeed for much of the journey I was asleep. Mum told me years later that we drove past the Sydney Opera House along the way, yet I myself didn't notice it.

But on the other hand I was very fascinated with the way the windshield wipers were making a pattern of water on the glass while it was raining. I couldn't understand how the wipers were able to work without a person moving them, and the patterns of rain left on the glass (where the wipers didn't reach) interested me a great deal. The place which caught my attention most was the triangular shape of wet glass left between the two wipers at the bottom of the windshield.

During the trip I also remember stopping by an open grass field in a park, where the adults of my family socialised and had lunch and dinner. By the late evening I became both tired and bored, and that caused me to have a tantrum. Mum took me back to the car where I could finish crying. It didn't take too long for me to calm down enough to see what my mother was holding in her hand. The object was what I now know to be a tennis ball and she handed it to me saying that I could keep it. This tennis ball remained a favourite sensory item until I was seven years old, when it was sadly ripped apart by our pet dog.

As I further approached my second birthday, I spent much more time outside on the verandah, or in my sandpit which was in the corner of our back garden. While I was in the sandpit I almost always wore my swimwear (even though I wasn't going for a swim) and I simply loved to play with the sand. This may at first glance seem like a very lame statement.

However the sand itself was so much more than just simple fun. Its very texture was coarse and therapeutic to squeeze with my hands, and it also had a fascinating and pleasing smell. I hadn't ever experienced the smell of wet sand, of the kind that we sense whenever we tip a bucket of that substance over to create a sandcastle. As a toddler I realised that damp sand could stick together to create so many things. That to me was truly magical, and still is now to some extent.

Soon the mornings were getting much warmer as December came nearer, and being able to walk more successfully meant that I would leave my bedroom a fair while prior to breakfast. While my mother was busy in the kitchen she would give me a large poster (printed on cardboard) of all the letters of the alphabet and the numbers up to nine. At that time I did not know in any way how to read and understand the concept of letters and numbers. But I entertained myself by making up words for each one of them I saw.

Also, whenever I saw the letter 'P' I said "parking spot", because we lived in the inner city (where I had seen that symbol many times during car trips to the shops) and my parents would say those words almost every time they saw a small sign with the letter 'P'. Whilst I was in the company of adults having conversations, I could not understand everything they were saying. However I would pick out odd words here and there, particularly if they were brief and repetitive. Even to this very day, I continue to use this exact same method whilst I'm learning languages other than English. In my own opinion it's the most effective way to quickly advance one's general vocabulary, pronunciation and ability to form sentences.

As my year of (mostly) being a two year old approached, there was also set to be yet another life changing event, that would give me an important reason to mature. At the age of one, I could not at all predict the occurrence of this upcoming change. But I received a shock when the event came along, and I had no choice other than to accept it.

CHAPTER THREE

LIFE IS NOT THE SAME FOR ME ANYMORE

When my second birthday came along many people came to see me (just like they had done on my previous birthday), and I had a cake with a toy train on top and some tinsel wrapped around the side of it. After I'd blown out the candles and the cake was cut, I kept the plastic train and it was my favourite toy for several months afterward.

At that young age I had no idea that my parents were expecting another child, and my biological sister, Jessica, was born on January the 7th, 1992. For almost a whole year I hadn't paid any attention whatsoever to my mother's growing stomach, and of course at such a young age I didn't yet know that children begin their lives in the womb. Yes, I myself had began life in my mother's womb as well. Though my view of mum being pregnant with me could only possibly be from the inside of her.

On that day my parents explained to me that Jessica was my sister and that this second child would be added to the family. Though I still didn't understand and was more interested in playing with my toy train.

The next year required a fair bit of adjustment for me. This was because another child was getting equal attention, and not all of the toys in the house were solely my own anymore. As well, I had to learn how to take turns with other things, such as watching television. Then additionally all of the toys that I had outgrown were passed down to Jessica. Despite the fact that I didn't play with them anymore, I still remembered how much I had previously liked them. Memories of me enjoying those toys always resurfaced whenever I saw them, so I strongly felt as if she was stealing my property!

There was also a time when me and Jessica were watching television together. I was sat on some pillows on the floor, and Jessica was in her pram. When my parents had left the room I mischievously wheeled Jessica into her bedroom and came back to watch television on my own. At that age we think that we're so much cleverer than we really are. Mum came into the living room, looking straight at me and asked "Where's your sister, Rebecca"? I then answered "The baby wanted to look at her bedroom". Amusingly I still mistakingly believed that my mother would never know what I actually did!

Additionally, my anxiety of sleeping at nighttime continued, and this would cause me to do other mischievous things. If I woke up when my parents were still awake, I would climb out of bed and deliberately start knocking my toys around. The noise would always bring my mother into the room.

So I would then spend an hour or so in the living room with my parents until I felt tired and safe. Whilst in the living room, I would usually go on my rocking horse until I had no energy left, and would then say "I want to go back to bed now". The rocking horse was an excellent sleep remedy for me at that time, and I would be encouraged by my parents to rock as fast as I possibly could!

On the other hand, if I woke up early in the morning, my mother would continue to give me an alphabet book to look at, so that I could entertain myself instead of waking everybody else up. Something else which I enjoyed reading was the street directory. I definitely would have loved Google Earth and Google Street View if it had existed back then.

By that time I had experienced enough car trips to understand how they meant that we were going somewhere. The first time mum handed me the street directory to look at, she told me that the lines were the roads of which we traveled. As a two year old I had some understanding (yet not as much as today) of how those lines symbolised our streets.

My mother also began giving me various kinds of lessons during the day, when it was just me and her at home. Jessica was at home too, but she was asleep in her crib. The sort of activities mum would give me mainly involved drawing, colouring in and reading books. There was a time when I was given a picture of a dog to colour in with a packet of crayons. However I couldn't understand all of the words mum would say to me during those moments, despite being very interested in figuring out what she was telling me.

There was a lesson when I was holding a blue crayon, and instinctively I put the crayon to the paper and started to colour all over it. My mother kept saying "No, stay in the lines". In truth I did not understand the meaning of any of those words back then. Yet purely by luck, my mother then said "That's it, you're right" when I eventually began colouring the section where she was guiding my hand.

Jigsaw puzzles would also entertain me, and once I got bored with repeatedly putting together the same pictures, I would turn the pieces over and put them together with the plain cardboard/wooden side (without the printed picture) facing upward. To this day I still thoroughly enjoy putting together both tangible and digital jigsaw puzzles.

There are other kinds of puzzles which I enjoy too, such as solving Rubik's Cubes of various sizes and logic puzzles, particularly those involving process of elimination and cracking codes. Many years later (as an adult) it was discovered via an adaptive functioning test that this was my 'spark area', and for cracking codes I scored in the 99th percentile. The reason for me later having an adaptive functioning test was because I eventually would receive a diagnosis of autism.

But the age of two was the time when my ASD (Autism Spectrum Disorder) characteristics began to show in a very significant way. I'd spend much more time organising the cutlery drawer into forks and spoons than I did by playing with my age appropriate toys. I'd also get highly distressed if my routine was changed. Hugging and showing people affection were aspects of life which were (and still are) unnatural to me as well.

Once, I was standing in the living room and I looked up at mum, who suddenly threw out her arms (as a gesture of her wanting to hug me). But until I was told, I didn't know why she had done that action. Though mum told me that it was for her to give me a cuddle and that she was quite upset that I seemingly refused. At this I burst into tears and tried to tell her (with my limited two year old vocabulary) that I didn't mean to upset her. It was purely because I didn't understand what her nonverbal gesture was. But even so, there was much more in regards to spending time with mum, that didn't involve physical gestures such as hugging.

Throughout that year I would enjoy being in the kitchen with my mother whenever she was preparing meals. She would occasionally get me to help her with simple things like stirring the cake mixture. There was one time when I picked up a bowl (even though mum told me not to), put my whole face into it, had a good smell of the chopped onions, and then rubbed a large piece directly into my eyes. They stung and watered for about fifteen minutes, and I haven't done that twice!

I'd often like to help mum as a way of being kind, though at times I feel that it was more a case of me being able to prove that I could do more 'grown up' stuff!

Though I still thoroughly enjoyed doing 'kids stuff' as well. Hence the reason why I spent a lot of time sat down at my own plastic child size table with my jumbo sized crayons. To be honest I didn't like the smell of the crayons whenever I used them. However the way that they could bring pictures to life with colour mostly made up for that.

There were many other times when I'd be sat down using my crayons and my mother would tell me to do things, such as cleaning away mess on my floor, getting dressed to go out or having to go to bed when it was time. Constantly I would say the word "later" and my mother would respond with "now". Yet getting told off was something that really upset me. Whenever Mum said "I'm very disappointed with you, Becky", I would say "Later disappointed, Mummy", and would press two fingers against her lips with tears in my eyes. This sensation of guilt would always enable me to do as my mother asked. Though a mere couple months after then, another upsetting event occurred for me.

In November of 1992 my parents divorced and for the next few months we lived at my grandparents' house. Our stay there was very brief, though there are still many recollections of personal significance. There was a time (during the month of moving in) when I was walking across the driveway and I tripped over some gravel near the front door. I fell down and grazed my knee, and grazes hurt so much more when we are a two/three year old, compared to how they do as an adult. Memories of that incident bring an 'echo' of the pain back to my left knee. Nowadays I don't even notice any grazes I get. Yet back then it stung so badly that it made my eyes water.

It's incredible how our perspective of things like pain change so much as we grow older and more mature. My best guess as to why this is the case for me is perhaps due to the fact that I've since been grazed and bruised so often throughout all the years. Therefore maybe I have now become more desensitised to such minor pains.

Hence the reason why I now wish that I could give the words of "if you think a graze hurts just be prepared for next year's injury" to my two/three year old self, if I could travel back to November of 1992.

CHAPTER FOUR

ADJUSTING TO LIFE WITHIN A FAMILY OF THREE PEOPLE

On my third birthday I still didn't know what the day meant, and was surprised when my mother placed a strawberries and cream cake in front of me. When she said "this is for you", I misunderstood and picked off a strawberry as I was all set to eat it myself. However she told me that it was indeed my cake but it was for me to *share* with my family and friends.

Two weeks later mum woke me up to say that Santa had been. At that time I had no knowledge of calendar dates and couldn't yet piece together the concept of getting presents on Christmas Day; nor did I yet have the childhood belief of Santa Claus arriving overnight to deliver them.

On that Christmas morning it was very early and I didn't really feel like following my mother out into the living room, as I was still rather groggy. However I woke up immediately when I saw heaps of new toys and my mother said "They're all yours". These included a Baby Alive doll which I played with until breakfast. Though once mum had taken me and Jessica outside to see our 'big present', which was a new swing set, I spent the rest of the day out on the patio.

A little while later I had one of my early vaccinations. Up until I was almost in my teen years I was terrified of getting needles. I absolutely hated the anticipation of the pinprick and the sting of the liquid being injected. Though despite the pain, mum would always promise me an affordable treat afterward, which would either be some candy or a small toy. After I had come home from a vaccination (at the age of three), I had a very interesting and memorable conversation with my mother.

At three years old I would ask mum many questions relating to experiences I had years or months beforehand. Mum's constant reply to me was "I don't know Becky, it was a long time ago". There was a moment where my mother said this again while I was sat on a bed at my grandparents' house (after the vaccination that I mentioned above). It was then when I said "But one day right *now* will be a long time ago". Mum smiled and then said "Yes, and when that time comes you won't remember it". This has now become an amusing topic of discussion.

After living at our grandparents' house for a few months we eventually moved into a small townhouse. This was the beginning of a long phase of our life when it was just the three of us living together (me, Jessica and our mother). As a family we would do many fun things, such as going to Dreamworld (one of our local theme parks) time and time again.

Yet there were many more significant things that shaped the person who I am today. By the age of three, I had extreme anxiety along with depression. Sleeping was still a frightening activity for me. However I now had the verbal skills to ask my mother "Why do you keep taking us out to all of these weird places every night"? This was when mum told me that those nighttime adventures were dreams, and that dreams are made up by our mind. She also told me that it was my mind who took me out on those nighttime ventures, and only my mind could wake me up.

Initially, as a three year old I misunderstood this, and believed that 'mind' was a person. For instance, there was a dream I had (which was lucid as usual) where I was in an unfamiliar environment and wanted to wake up. So I asked every dream character where 'mind' was, and how I wished to speak to him.

Eventually I was told that 'mind' was behind a closed door that I was lead to, and that he *did* want to speak to me. Once the door opened however, I received a slight surprise. It seemed that I was all alone in a dark room and was facing what looked like a black bowling ball.

Though immediately this ball disassembled itself (very much like a Transformers character) and then all of the nuts and bolts reassembled themselves into the shape of a human face.

After the moment of me being startled passed, I finally asked Mind if

I could wake up. Yet he told me that I must never be scared of dreams, and that while I'm dreaming I can experience absolutely anything I wish for when I'm awake. This is what my mother had previously told me.

Mind then informed me that rather than trying to wake up from dreams I don't like, I should change them into something that I find happy or exciting instead.

But then I told him that my mother had said that only he could control my dreams. Yet his reply before I finally woke up was "But I am you". Then in answer to my puzzled look he said "You are Mind".

When I told my mother about this dream the next day she said that my mind was a part of me, which I had full control over. She said (in three year old language) that its existence and appearance resides in all of my thoughts, feelings and imagination. Therefore the reason for Mind's strange appearance was a result of what I imagined him to look like. It was the same story for the rest of my dream as well.

So I finally understood that dreams weren't real (in a physical sense) and that took much of the fear away. Though nightmares still scared me, especially those which involved me being taken away from my mum, and when there were great big monsters. At that stage the monsters of my dreaming imagination were everyday objects that all of a sudden came alive, grew teeth and chased me around until they bit me.

Sometimes those monsters were initially disguised as objects, including a cup I was holding or a chair I would be sitting in. Fortunately I was able to force myself to wake up before I got 'bitten', however I still found the experience of being chased very frightening. During that time I was going through a bad phase of nightmares and this was one of the main reasons as to why my mother took me to see a psychiatrist.

Mum expressed that in addition to my anxiety she also believed that I had autism. This was because I didn't socialise too well, would get highly distressed if my routine changed, would refuse to cuddle anybody, and would scream if someone brushed past me. However the psychiatrist (who was still kind and very helpful to me over the years) didn't believe that this was related to autism and felt that it was all related to my parents' divorce. This was primarily due to how little was understood or documented about autism back in 1993. I continued to receive psychotherapy throughout my childhood and teenage years. Yet I wasn't diagnosed with autism until I was fifteen years old. More of that will be mentioned in a later chapter.

But so many other memorable events happened in my life before then. Say, there was an occasion when I was three years old (and Jessica was one year old), and Mum would have both me and her sat down at our plastic table outside for lunch. Though for a short while, I got up to quite some mischief during the moments when our mother was inside (before I quickly and easily got caught). As I was three years old and my sister was one, I could walk and use my hands so much better than she could. Taking full advantage of that, I would quickly pick up Jessica's plate of food as soon as mum walked inside (whilst she was keeping an eye on us through the window) and toss it into the bushes. Then I would hurry back to my seat to finish my own meal.

If I were to observe this childish activity purely from an adult perspective, I would probably read it as sibling rivalry and a desire to make my baby sister starve. Though that wasn't the actual reason. Back then I merely thought it was a clever and funny way to show off my dexterity skills, and I didn't feel like this cruel action mattered, as long as it wasn't my own meal.

Yet mum caught me out by noticing that after less than sixty seconds I had a full plate of food, while Jessica's plate was empty. Clearly I wasn't as clever as I then felt I was, and mum solved the problem by getting me to swap plates with Jessica. It was then when I learned my lesson and never tossed her lunch away again.

While we're on the subject of food, later that year there was also a time when I had a dream, where I was being taken around a building with my mother. We walked past a cafe selling cakes and biscuits. So I kept pleading for some by wailing "chocolate cookies" to my mum. Her repeated response was "we haven't got any". Funnily enough I woke myself up by shouting "chocolate cookies" and mum said "for the last time Becky, we don't have any"! I didn't realise that I was actually saying those words out loud while I was sleeping.

There was another event that occurred in 1993 which was far less humorous. It was when I had my first surgical operation in a hospital.

CHAPTER FOUR

One day I was playing in the living room and tripped over a rug. That made me fall face forward into the corner of a coffee table. Unluckily the place where I deeply cut myself happened to be on a large vein just beneath my eyebrow. So my face was covered with blood and I was crying.

Mum called the paramedics immediately and I was taken to Logan Hospital. Though we got told that I'd have to be transferred to the Mater Children's Hospital (which has now been expanded and is reffered to as the Queensland Children's Hospital), due to where the cut was and the kind of surgery that was required. So they patched me up quickly and then I was carried into an ambulance once again. Mum then explained to me that I was being taken to a different hospital.

While I was there it was quite scary for me. I was in a ward with about a dozen other children under the age of five. Despite not being told about the operation procedure or the fact that I would need anaesthesia, I was still very nervous about what was happening. All of the chaos and unfamiliarity gave me an intense amount of fear and Mum wasn't able to be present during the operation.

So I cried and screamed loudly as I was being wheeled down the corridors. The surgeons and doctors kept saying to me "Stop crying now. It's only going to make things worse". While I was in the operating room they told me to just lie down and take some deep breaths. They said that this 'magic medicine' would calm me down and make everything better. I fully believed them and then did what I was told to do.

Later that night I woke up in a comfortable bed in the ward. I still wasn't at home but I noticed that I had my loved ones around me, and I felt a large bandage on my face. My mother and the nurses told me that my eyebrow was stitched up and was unable to be touched for a while. A fair few weeks later I had my stitches removed and I screamed during that procedure too, as I didn't like the sensation of my skin being pinched and pulled.

Now as an adult I still have a deep scar under my left eyebrow after that accident. Mum got told by the surgeon in 1993 (without me being present) that if it bothered me when I got older, plastic surgery would be able to hide the scar.

But personally, I now feel that all that trouble and money just isn't worth it. In fact by the time I got to my teenage years I felt happy about having a scar on my forehead, as well as having to wear glasses because it was relatable to the fictional character Harry Potter. In later chapters you will read a great deal more about *Harry Potter*'s influence on my life.

During the following year (at the age of four), I would unexpectedly have to be in hospital again. But at the very least, my family and I learned a few things from my previous experience in 1993. So the next hospital visit wasn't anywhere near as stressful for me.

CHAPTER FIVE

I'M NOW FEELING
READY TO GROW UP

In December of 1993 I had my fourth birthday. I still didn't understand what the meaning of that day was. But it made me so happy to unwrap a pair of roller-skates and a helmet in the morning. Later that evening my grandparents came to visit, and brought along a toy makeup kit as well as a dollhouse.

For a short while I enjoyed smelling the scented makeup and putting it on as if it were face paint. But eventually it started to make my skin itch (I've always had those kinds of allergies) and I had to wash it all off. Afterward my attention wandered off to the dollhouse which I played with for much longer. I was particularly fascinated by the electric light in its living room.

Over and over again I would be entertained by turning the light off and on. To me, at that age it felt as if I were a giant who was managing a real house, which was so small that some of the rooms could be taken over by my whole hand! In my imagination my hand was a person, and I would perform a 'walking' action with my middle and index fingers.

Two weeks later was Christmas Day and that was a very similar experience. We unwrapped our presents in the living room, which was a toy kitchen for me and a toy washing machine for Jessica. The morning was spent by us playing with those toys. Though for the rest of the day we got to skate outside on the patio. This entertained me until night came, despite the pavement area and garden being so small.

Throughout the next year (which was 1994) Mum would take me and Jessica to Dreamworld every weekend. Jessica and I would be entertained by the same two shows each and every time. There was a show where puppets would sing songs which me and my sister would re-enact while doing 'Dreamworld Shows' at home, even though we got most of the lyrics wrong.

But our favourite show would have to have been watching Kenny and Belinda Koala (the park's two character mascots) and The Gum Nut Fairy (who is no longer featured today).

It began with a magic show which I didn't fancy as much due to the balloons and loud bangs. To this day the sound of balloons bursting (as well as fireworks, guns and explosions with a similar sound) has remained to be my worst fear. Due to this phobia there have been some very embarrassing experiences over the years, which include me fainting (from intense fear) during a show at another theme park.

But afterwards the two 'koalas' and the fairy hosted a dance show where random kids from the crowd were given free ice-cream vouchers. Jessica and I had been attending that show weekly for several months and we weren't initially being picked for a prize. As a four year old that made me very upset. But after several months of attending that show, my sister and I were eventually getting picked regularly from the audience.

It all began when I started wearing a sparkly multicoloured sequin cap that was given to me by my grandparents. Kenny and Belinda liked this hat very much and whilst I was on stage they asked me where I had bought it.

I answered by saying that we had visited the South Bank markets a short time beforehand, and we walked past a stall selling some essentials for the beach. Grandad asked me if I would prefer a bucket and spade or the colourful hat that I had spotted, and I decided that what I truly wanted was the hat. Ironically this hat stayed with me for roughly ten years and every time I wore it I got plenty of compliments. This even included a moment when I wore the cap in a school play during my early high school years. So it remained stylish well into the 2000s.

Though returning to my personal recollections from the year 1994, the hit Disney film *The Lion King* was released a short time after my first stage appearance with the sparkly hat. Of the two of us Jessica was the one who was most excited to see it, but I too looked forward to the excitement of going to the cinema. Nowadays cinemas seem like large living rooms to me. But up until my preteen years, going to the movies was as exciting as going on a holiday.

After seeing the movie, we went into the foyer to 'meet' the life-size cardboard cutouts of various Disney characters. Jessica was trying to hug each and every one of them while mum took some pictures. Yet I was so overwhelmed by the whole experience that I tended to edge behind the figures in the photos. Mum interpreted this as shyness. But the truth was that I was fascinated by the fact that these 'people' and 'animals' were flat at the back, and that they didn't truly exist in living form.

There was another time when my mother made a false assumption that I was being shy. This was when we went to see a Johnson and Friends concert. Johnson and Friends was a children's television show that had many similarities to Disney Pixar's *Toy Story*. The toys came alive whenever their child owner, Michael was asleep or not present. Not all of the characters were toys either. For instance there was a hot water bottle and even a banana peel! Anyhow, me and Jessica brought along our plush toys of Johnson the elephant and McDuff the concertina.

A newspaper photographer came by to take a picture of us holding our toys. But neither me nor Jessica had any idea what it all meant. At that moment I saw the doors to the concert open and I sprinted to the auditorium afraid that I'd miss the show. Jessica meanwhile stayed behind long enough for a picture to be taken of her.

Another part of my life which puzzles me is that for some very strange reason I have frequently found myself being given requests for media stories. This has been happening unexpectedly throughout my life whenever I've been in the most random of places. I have no idea why this is the case because I'm definitely not celebrity material. Yet somehow it has always happened, and I only realised about how unusual this is when one of the producers of our family's 2022 documentary film mentioned it recently.

That year (in 1994) Mum also decided that it would be good for us to do dance classes as a hobby. She felt that we would enjoy them as we liked doing performances and wearing costumes at home. Initially Mum decided upon ballet for Jessica who she's always felt that she is the one who is more 'arty', mainly in regards to the way she dresses and moves. Whereas Mum's first choice for me was to try out jazz dancing, and if I didn't like it I could do ballet with Jessica. Personally I found jazz dancing too fast paced and I didn't like the punk-rock music which I had to dance too. So I ended up doing ballet for a short while because the classical music was soothing and calming. Listening to classical music has continued to be a relaxing daily activity for me.

On a somewhat bleaker note, in 1994 I also had my second operation in a hospital, this time for the removal of my tonsils and adenoids. Strangely when I got tonsillitis, I didn't feel that unwell as I had always had issues with allergies. The only difference was that my throat was a lot more painful than usual. Though when I woke up one morning, Mum looked at me sympathetically and said "You're not well at all are you". She then mentioned, in four year old language, that the results had come back from the doctor and I would have to go to hospital for an operation.

Mum knew that my last hospital visit was very stressful for me, and she wanted to find a place in which I would feel more comfortable. So I had my operation at the Sunnybank Private Hospital instead of the Mater Children's Hospital. Prior to having my operation later that night, I built a Lego house with a couple of boys who were in the same ward as me.

This put me into a relaxed state so that I wasn't screaming all the way down the corridors, as had been the case a year before. In the early hours of the morning I woke up in the ward where all of the children's beds were. I felt comforted when I saw my family standing around me, despite noticing that there was a drip attached to my left hand. Mum told me that I had just had my tonsils and adenoids taken out and I couldn't eat anything for a few hours, despite the fact that I was very hungry (given that I hadn't eaten for over twelve hours). My grandmother and Aunt told me that they too had their tonsils removed in their early childhood. I was also assured that I was very brave, because they remembered how painful and scary the experience was for them.

I had to take a few weeks off daycare after that operation. Though the time came when I had to return. Nap time was always difficult for me because I had trouble sleeping during the daytime. There was never a time when I slept, as I wanted to play with the toys (though not with other children) and/or go for a walk.

One day while the supervisor was in her office, I sneaked out of the room and walked over to the window of the next room where the older children were. They were awake and making paper butterflies and gluing cellophane to their wings. The supervisor of that room then saw me and I braced myself, as I thought that I'd get into trouble for being out of bed and having crept out of my supervisor's sight.

Though the young woman greeted me with a smile and said "Hello there, would you like to come in? We're making butterflies. Do you want to make one too"? The main thought that was on my mind was that I was so glad to be doing this instead of struggling to fall asleep on the floor.

While I got into the process of the activity, it kept me entertained until my mother picked me up later that afternoon. When Mum walked in she was accompanied by the supervisor who I had sneaked away from in the previous room. They were both very pleased that I had (by my own free will) decided to move into a room with kids who were slightly more advanced age wise. I was also told that I could remain in the 'big kids room' permanently as I was then four years old and willing to mature.

Up until very recently children in Queensland began school the year when they turned six. This meant that I was officially due to start Grade 1 in January 1995, even though I would not turn six until December.

However both my mother and my preschool teacher didn't feel I was ready to start school, despite how excited and eager I felt about it. Their opinion was that a child who turned five a month before the year started (our school year begins in January and ends in December) was too young, and especially given that I was a particularly young five year old socially and emotionally. Indeed, if I were to have been born a mere three weeks later, I wouldn't have been able to start school until 1996 anyhow. So the decision was for me to start school the following year instead, and remain attending the daycare centre in the meantime.

CHAPTER SIX

A NEW HOUSE TO ALWAYS CALL HOME

My fifth birthday was the first time when I knew what the day meant, and that I had counted the days down to. Early that morning I had run into my mother's bedroom shouting that the day had finally arrived. She then accompanied me down into the living room where I opened my presents. I had been given a new Disney sleeping bag, along with a radio and a cassette player. Millennials were the generation who began their lives with CDs and cassette tapes, and then in our preteen/teenage years iPods and streaming apps (for music and films) were increasingly available.

We spent most of my birthday that year at Dreamworld where I had such an amazing time. I even got to have a ride through the park in Kenny and Belinda's van and the Gum Nut Fairy sang Happy Birthday to me on stage during the show. In the evening we arrived home, had some birthday cake and then it was time for bed. As a treat, my sister and I got to sleep out in the living room instead of our bedrooms. I slept in my new sleeping bag and dozed off while listening to a Disney audiobook, which was *101 Dalmatians*.

Perhaps most importantly however, the following year (1995) was when we moved into the house that we are currently living in now. Our initial house was a rented home that was temporary for us. But that year Mum was set to get a house which was newly built and a place which would have belonged to us from the beginning. Mum got us so excited about moving into our new place, and we had a fair few visits to the construction site, from the moment when it was being built from the foundation.

Though it did make me feel sad one night as I was trying to fall asleep in my old bedroom. It was by the sudden thought that this bedroom would no longer be my safe haven, and that it would end up belonging to a stranger. From where I lay that night I heard the sound of mum's television coming up from downstairs. I couldn't hear the voices of the people talking too clearly. Yet from a combination of imagination and hearing them from a distance, I was listening to a family talking about their home belonging to them and no one else. In my imagination these were the next people who would live in *our* house and in *my* bedroom.

Yet when the time came for me to move my furniture and toys into my new bedroom I felt a sense of excitement, and all of those previous feelings of possessiveness were then lost.

It was every weekend when mum would take us to see our new home being built. On Saturday afternoons after ballet class we would have McDonalds for lunch, as a treat for while we were sitting in our almost fully built bedrooms.

On the night prior to us finally moving in we stayed at mum's sister's house, which was a two minute drive from where we were about to live. The next morning Jessica and I were welcomed home by our mother and two pet cats, Clancy and Ambrose. When I was shown into my new bedroom all of my furniture had been assembled and placed, as had all of my toys.

As a five year old, I mostly understood that a very time consuming job had been done for me, and I was pleased. However I didn't at all understand just how *stressful* moving between houses actually was for the adults. My understanding at five was that the task would be more or less like tidying my room was.

As well, I didn't appreciate the fact that the furniture of all the other rooms of the house (in addition to those in my bedroom) had been placed and assembled within a mere couple of nights!

A few weeks after moving into our new home however, something very upsetting happened. One morning before going to daycare we couldn't find my cat Ambrose anywhere. Mum hoped that she hadn't gotten lost or been in a terrible accident. She told me that we should wait a few days until Ambrose came home.

Though she never did. After a month I was still hopeful that Ambrose would come back. But mum said "She won't come back sweetie. She's run away, and probably has a new home now". At that age I interpreted those words as meaning that Ambrose had found another home and family to live with.

However a short while after accepting the disappointing truth, our mother asked me and Jessica at dinner time one evening about how we'd feel about getting a new pet dog. She said that the puppy would be my new pet as I had just lost Ambrose.

I was slightly scared of dogs back then because I had heard words of caution at daycare about dogs biting kids if they were annoyed. Though the idea of a new pet still excited me.

The next week mum took me and Jessica out to collect our puppy. By that time I felt a mixture of excitement and fear. Though once I saw the puppy she didn't look scary at all. She was a spoodle (cocker spaniel/poodle cross) and looked so cute and harmless. Mum decided to call her Sparky. After collecting Sparky we visited our grandparents' house and let her have a wander around. In those days they used to dock the tails of certain dogs, thus Sparky was excitedly wagging a tail about the length of my (current) index finger.

Mum also had a tin of what we were told was the puppy's favourite brand of dog food, which was called 'Pal'. As soon as mum put Sparky's dish on the concrete floor in the laundry, she ate up all of the food in less than a minute, with her little tail wagging away as she did so.

By the time we finally got home and were ready for bed Mum said that Sparky was to sleep with her that night. She also told me and Jessica to not be so loud around her, as she was only a puppy and would get scared. Though when mum wasn't looking I got this rather mean idea of testing a boundary.

When Sparky came into my dark bedroom through the open door (as she was allowed to walk around the house until mum went to bed), I jumped out of bed and roared at her with a monster face. Poor Sparky whimpered, and at the time I thought that it was the sound she would always make instead of a bark. Prior to having one as a pet I had only ever heard of dogs making one sound, which was a bark.

However roughly a month afterward it was my own turn to be scared in the same way as poor Sparky was. To this day I have a chronic sleep condition called Sleep Paralysis Disorder, where if I don't take Anafranil (a form of medication) daily I experience nightly problems. Having Sleep Paralysis Disorder means that it takes a while for my brainwaves to shift instantly between REM (Rapid Eye Movement) Sleep and wakefulness. So I will either be paralysed for up to a few minutes after waking up or I will have a night terror, where my mind will continue dreaming for a short time after my eyes open.

At the age of five I had a particularly frightening night terror (that occurred when my eyes were open yet I was still halfway through a dream) which has continued to be on my mind to this very day. There was a morning when I had just opened my eyes and I heard a rattling noise beside my bed. I turned around and saw a red shapeless monster (which resembled the evil Jafar shooting out of his genie lamp in Aladdin) zoom towards me with a roar.

I was extremely scared and I couldn't sleep in my own bedroom for almost a year, because at the time I genuinely believed that a monster lived in there. To make matters even worse, a sadistic adult had previously told me a story about monsters (names oo-na-nas) living in the ceilings of children's bedrooms, and coming out at night to hurt them while they were in bed.

After hearing the story of my 'red monster dream', this adult told me that what I saw really was an 'oo-na-na' and that I should have listened to him when he told me they were real. So after that experience I knew just how the puppy had felt when I had cruelly scared her.

On a much more positive note, in the latter half of 1995 our mother had finally added a sandpit to our garden. This made me and Jessica very happy as we had a new playground to build things in; and it made mum happy because she no longer had to clean away the mess from us building sandcastles and trenches in the dirt and mud. There was a time shortly before we got a sandpit when us kids thought that it would be fun to cover ourselves from head to toe in mud!

But it wasn't so fun when our mother said "Look at the state of you both! Stand over there so I can hose you down, and then take yourselves into the bathroom for a wash"! I didn't like the sensation of having to be hosed down all over, and I felt much more like playing than having a bath. It's true that we did have toys in the bath. Yet they weren't nearly as much fun as our other things to play with were. Thus another idea of messy play that I initially thought would be enjoyable, was taken off my list for the future.

Shortly afterward, in November of 1995 I experienced my first ever concert for my ballet class. Me and my fellow 5/6 year old dancers were dressed as yellow fairies with butterfly wings. Mum still has that costume stored away, and I was very happy to keep all of my other costumes for several years to come as well.

The first time I saw my costume for the Pollyanna themed concert was when I woke up in the early hours of the morning (from a loud thunderstorm), and mum cheered me up by getting me to try it on.

I was unable to attend the previous year's concert in 1994, but I had heard so many positive things about it. Yet after attending my first concert in 1995, I realised just how exciting they truly were. While we were backstage waiting for our performance we were also each given a giant cookie to eat. We were of course brushed clean of crumbs just prior to going on stage.

A month later, I thoroughly enjoyed my 6th birthday at our new house. December the 11th fell on a Monday in 1995, but we did the big celebration on the 10th instead. This was because I was set to have a busy enough day on the Monday with other activities. However Mum did say to me "If you open all of your presents today you'll have none to open tomorrow". But of course at that age I wanted to open everything as soon as possible.

Though I must admit I was a little furious with myself when I didn't have any presents left to unwrap on my actual birthday. I spent much of that day at preschool and I had a huge birthday cake which was the flavour of white chocolate, so it was very sweet indeed!

That afternoon was a balmy night in Brisbane with a late thunderstorm. While the thunder was rolling my nana suggested that I should start writing a journal to take note of the weather on each of my birthdays, and from there she gave me a suggestion of keeping a diary.

Despite having tried countless times to keep a diary, I have never succeeded. Handwriting feels awkward for me and I've always felt that it saves so much energy to just take note of events in my mind, rather than having my hand ache for no reason.

Later that evening I had my ballet end of year break-up party. The reason I was given such a large birthday cake was so we could take the leftovers along to the party. Everyone was also able to sing to me and wish me Happy Birthday while I was there. So it was a fabulous way to end what has remained to be my favourite date of each and every year.

SECTION TWO

STRUGGLES WITH AUTISM

CHAPTER SEVEN

SCHOOL IS NOT AS GREAT AS I THOUGHT IT WOULD BE

I did have autism right from the very beginning of my life, and was finally diagnosed with ASD as a fifteen year old. But for so many years I struggled with no assistance in regards to autism itself. The reason for why I got diagnosed in the year 2005 was because that was the time when more was being discovered about the feminine characteristics of autism. Autism actually affects both genders equally. Though traditionally more boys and men got diagnosed with autism, as the medical criteria was based almost entirely on its masculine characteristics.

It was also discovered that when a female would share the key characteristics of autism with boys and men (as many, if not most of the characteristics are the same regardless of gender) it would often get misdiagnosed as being an anxiety disorder and/or another psychiatric condition. That unfortunately was the case with myself.

Despite having enjoyed my childhood overall, the fact that my autism was diagnosed relatively late has had a huge impact on my adult life. Yet I will mention in later chapters how I now look back and am actually quite thankful for the lessons those challenges have taught me. I'll begin this chapter from the time when I was six years old (my first year at school), and gradually work my way forward to my early teenage years.

When I started Grade 1 at Boronia Heights State Primary School I had all the traits of an autistic child. If this would have been 2016 instead of 1996 I would most probably have been identified as having autism in an instant.

On the night before my very first school day I could hardly sleep from excitement. I felt so grown up about beginning school and was full of the typical childhood naivety that every kind of life change is exciting, prior to us having to actually *take on* that change. However when I had finished my first school day, I ran to my mum in tears, saying how happy I was to be going back home.

Grade One is nothing like kindergarten (or prep as it's now called in Queensland). In school, children are required to always work to their best ability and to achieve the best possible marks, which are mainly presented as stickers in our early years of school. It's nothing like preschool or kindergarten where we're generally allowed to do our own thing, if ever we're feeling too tired or anxious about doing any set activity. Children are no longer allowed to have naps in Grade One, and that takes time for them to adjust to. We're also away from our parents for longer than we were previously, and are expected to concentrate for a longer duration at story time.

For the first half of that year I cried constantly while I was at school. I missed my mother and sister (Jessica) so much. It didn't take long for me to get bullied by other kids as a result of this. One of the other school teachers said to my own teacher "Next year I never want to end up with *that* child in my classroom".

This was within my earshot and it hurt me a lot. Though at the age of six it's quite difficult to stand up for yourself against an adult seven times your age.

During recess a few days after that remark, I realised that screaming and crying didn't solve situations. More rather it made everything multiple times worse. So from that moment on (until many years later) I went completely silent and withdrew myself from everybody. I'd sit alone during recess and many kids bullied me for this new demeanour as well.

There was a day when a girl walked up to me and said "Why have you gone all quiet now? It's really weird and I don't like it". She then asked me if I knew what a 'freak' was. When I shook my head the girl explained to me that it was a word used for people like myself, who were 'strange' and 'not normal'.

At that very moment, the same teacher who expressed that she didn't want me in her classroom told this girl how proud she was of a piece of homework that she had just handed in. After I had said "but this girl just called me a freak", her response was "she's just stating a fact, you are a freak".

I felt like bursting into tears, as I was so hurt and angry. But I didn't out of my fear of being called a cry-baby again. So as a six year old I used that same energy to act out instead. I deliberately drew on the carpet with a crayon. Afterward I was sent into a room next door where I kicked and threw things across the room, spat on the window and pulled faces at people who walked past.

Finally I was sent to the admin office and I had to wait there until my mother collected me. As well, the head principal of the school (who was always very kind) looked at me sadly and said "I'm very disappointed in you, Rebecca". Those were the exact words said to me by my mum when I was two years old and misbehaved. So that distant memory (four years seems to be a very long time when we're six) was resurfaced in my mind, and this made me cry.

Eventually my mother arrived at school to pick me up that afternoon, and the first thing she got told was that I was sent to the admin office, due to having lashed out. Despite being very angry about what was said to me by that girl and (especially) that teacher, she was still not at all pleased with my misbehaviour that day.

That afternoon I had an appointment with my psychiatrist, and usually mum bought us a McDonalds Happy Meal afterward. Though mum said I was to miss out that evening due to my behaviour. Mum also told me that if the school was unable to clean the crayon drawings off the carpet (which luckily wasn't the case), she would be paying for new carpet out of my pocket money. Nevertheless she did end up expressing to the admin how appalled she was that I was called a freak by a teacher, yet nothing whatsoever was done about it by the school.

There was never another school day where I acted out with that level of immature anger. So I went back to just completely withdrawing myself.

Throughout that year I was also very possessive and protective of my belongings, as well as anything I physically touched during the day. We later knew that the cause of this came from a combination of Obsessive Compulsive Disorder, Post Traumatic Stress Disorder and HSAM (which makes me excessively clingy when it comes to my physical, psychological and emotional possessions). For that reason I collected a great amount of rocks and twigs in my schoolbag. Whenever I lost one of my possessions from home I became absolutely distraught. These included simple items such as drink bottles. While we were on a class excursion to Seaworld I accidentally left my drink bottle on the bus. Our school used public buses then, so there was no way of getting the bottle back.

Owing to that I bawled my eyes out with tears, but was unable to explain the reason for me being so upset. I was later diagnosed with Obsessive Compulsive Disorder at the age of sixteen, and that now makes it fully clear as to why I felt that possessive.

Though one of the teachers that came along to assist us on the excursion could not understand why losing something as simple as a drink bottle would make a child react the way I did. She put it down to the possibility of my mother being abusive. As soon as I found out that she had made that assumption, I assured her again and again that my mum was a wonderful woman who I loved very much.

However one of mum's favourite memories (of which I have had recent conversations with her about) is from June of that year. We were at her parents' house having dinner, just before Jessica and I were to be taken out to the circus. But I was taking a long time to finish my meal. I then asked my mother if I could put salt on my lettuce, and she said that I couldn't because it wouldn't taste good. However while she wasn't looking I grabbed the salt and poured it onto my last lettuce leaf.

Mum was right, it tasted absolutely disgusting. Though I was determined to keep a straight face, and hide any sign of shuddering when I was made to eat it up. Ironically I never admitted to mum that I had done what she had told me not to do until I was an adult!

The year 1996 was also the time when I had my (first) medical assessment for autism. It was brought up by a psychotherapist (not the psychiatrist of whom I had been seeing since I three years old) that she believed that I had autism and Intellectual Impairment (IQ below 70).

I then got assessed by a child psychologist who said that my IQ appeared to be above average (now my overall IQ been assessed as being 121 via a WAIS test) and that she didn't believe that I had autism. She stressed to my mother that autistic children are not able to form connections with anybody, and that the fact that I had a separation anxiety disorder with my mother proved that I wasn't autistic.

Though it was still acknowledged that I had high anxiety, which they thought was 100 percent related to Post Traumatic Stress Disorder. They also mistakingly believed that it was a phase that I'd outgrow. So I was given no extra assistance at school. However my regular therapy did continue, even though it wasn't at that time expected to be lifelong.

Aside from the difficulties mentioned, my first year of school wasn't a bad experience overall. I did indeed have many positive experiences at school in Grade One. Due to the separation anxiety issues I had with my mum, both her and my teacher agreed that it would be a good idea for her to spend some time in class with me each day, assisting with the lessons. This was to phase me into the procedure of school, and for me to gradually get used to not having my mum with me all day. It worked very well for me and by the end of the year I was fully able to attend school independently.

While mum was in class with me she would do fun activities (in relation to each specific lesson) with myself and the other children. I can remember her refilling the bottles of glue and her saying "Look kids, it looks like a volcano", when she slightly overfilled the bottle and it splashed a little onto the paper underneath. Mum would also do activities with us in regards to learning about coins and counting money. A fun activity we did was to have a coin underneath a piece of paper and then we would rub a crayon over the top, to reveal the coin beneath it. As a six year old I genuinely thought it was done by magic!

My teacher was also very pleased with the strength I had in spelling. Countless times I would correct her spelling on the board, and I always found it amusing whenever she spelled the word 'yacht' as 'yatch'. The teacher turned her head to mum on one occasion and sighed while saying "It's never good when a Grade One child corrects your spelling". Yet she wasn't disappointed with this, on the contrary the teacher was very impressed.

CHAPTER SEVEN

In addition to attending general school, I also was in dance school that year.

After my happy experience the previous year I was very excited to attend my ballet concert in November of 1996. The theme this time was *Mary Poppins*, and me and the rest of my class were dressed as bluebirds, dancing to the song 'Tuppence' from the film. As a relatively young child it was always a strange feeling to get positioned on stage in a room that looked much like a shed, and then immediately afterwards the curtains slowly opened to reveal an audience

But despite the strange feeling, I never experienced stage fright in front of an audience. In fact once the curtains opened I felt a rush of excitement within me. Now as an adult I experience this with my public talks. Just prior to being called up on stage I feel slightly nervous. Though once I'm actually on stage I feel relaxed, happy and animated. I've come to learn that it's all mind over matter!

Whilst I'm on the topic of personal confidence, I can also say that I psychologically grew in another area, as I moved towards my upcoming year of Grade Two at school. Throughout the next school year I was set to still have extreme anxiety. However I would no longer require my mother to be with me at school, and I would not be bullied nearly as much as I had been the previous year.

CHAPTER EIGHT

I'M A HAPPY CHILD BUT I DO HAVE CERTAIN FEARS AND PHOBIAS

At the end of 1996 I had my birthday during the last week of Grade One. It was a Wednesday and I woke up to a beautiful pink and gold sunrise. My presents included a DIY brick and mortar mini house (the size of a Lego set) and a plastic crown with sparkly jewels in it. I wore that crown to school and I brought a birthday cake to class.

A week later I had a birthday party at McDonalds and so many classmates came along to celebrate with me. As I was a quiet student Mum was initially surprised by this. However she was surprised in a delightful way.

On Christmas Day me and Jessica were given a heap of presents. Jessica was given an enormous wooden dollhouse, along with Barbie dolls and soft toys to play with. I myself was given a Vtech kid's laptop computer, a solar powered calculator, a Barbie doll dressed in a school uniform (which after a few years I completely damaged, regrettably), a refracting telescope and a toy microscope. Then, a few weeks later I began my next year of school.

Grade Two was very much like the previous year. At that time I developed an intense interest in atlases, flags of the world and capital cities. In class I'd write all of my short stories about visiting foreign countries that I had never been to but had read about. I learned the capital cities for each country, so obsessively that I still know them to this day. I would literally sleep with an atlas under my pillow. At home mum and I would do craft activities where we would make my favourite world flags out of fabric. I must add that the US flag was the hardest to make due to its fifty stars.

CHAPTER EIGHT

Another interest that I developed simultaneously was outer space. I gained a basic knowledge of our solar system and the universe beyond. A fascination of artificial satellites came along, and I built my own 1970s style satellite (a cardboard and aluminium foil version) to hang from my bedroom ceiling. Satellites and space probes have always fascinated me far more than shuttles, and as a child I desperately wanted to visit the Kennedy Space Centre sometime in my life. That finally happened when I was twenty one years old which I'll mention again in a later chapter.

That year was also the beginning of a new phobia that lasted a long time, which was about fire and of my house burning down. I was terrified of lighters, matches, open flames and everything electrical. Seeing a news story about a Brisbane City shop explosion in mid 1997 gave me several sleepless nights. Nowadays with my Sleep Paralysis Disorder I occasionally have night-terrors where I will see my bedroom in flames with smoke everywhere for a brief moment after opening my eyes. Yet once my mind is fully awake I realise that there was never anything wrong.

Another lifelong fear (of which I've mentioned previously) is of the sounds of explosions, pyrotechnics and balloons bursting. Whenever my class at school involved balloon games I would cry and scream. I felt extremely embarrassed and knew that it would create further issues with bullying. Yet I purely and simply couldn't stop myself. I'd also get petrified at school fetes, which would always have both balloons and fireworks. My class did an excursion to Movie World that year, and they were going to see a magic show. Both my mother and I told my teacher in private that I couldn't go due to my phobias. That was then settled and they were perfectly fine with that.

Despite not going to Movie World with my classmates that year, I did get to visit the theme park a few months later with mum and Jessica. As a family we had a local holiday on the Gold Coast. We stayed at Pelican Cove for a week and did some fishing, activities in books of which mum bought us (I myself chose maths and spelling books), swimming and visiting the local theme parks. We didn't do Dreamworld that time, but we did go to Sea World, Ice World and Movie World.

At Ice World we were in a gigantic freezer and got to see incredible sculptures and playground equipment carved out of ice, and we also got to play in some fake snow. Mum was disappointed because she just saw it as a mere freezer. Though as children me and Jessica excitedly felt like we had visited the North Pole! At that time I genuinely believed that I had finally seen and played in real snow.

When we visited Sea World, Jessica tried catching all of the 'fish' while we watched the 3D movie in the cinema, and we got to see the dolphins and orcas in their ponds too while watching the live shows. Movie World was fun as well, even though I did get scared a few times. Throughout the police academy stunt performance I screamed due to the loud bangs.

There was also a moment during a show featuring gremlins when everyone was told to "run and leave the place immediately". That was meant to be part of the show. However I took what they said literally and bolted through the back door, leaving all of my belongings in the theatre!

Mum, Jessica and a couple of the cast members followed me outside and gradually assured me that there was no real emergency. I was also handed back the things I dropped while running out of the building.

Nowadays if I had run out of a show screaming like this (and had been gullible enough to believe that the actors were being serious), it would have made me so embarrassed that I'd be unable to visit the park for several years. Though perhaps seven year old children are a little more immune to embarrassment. Indeed when I look back now there are a fair few memories I have which (literally) make me wince out loud, and I sincerely hope that I'm the only one who remembers those events!

Parts of Movie World that I did enjoy however were the Looney Toons river ride and the rest of Looney Toons village, the street parade and the shops on Main Street where I bought a plush Scooby Doo. I slept with that toy for several years afterward.

Another family outing that I enjoyed in (June) 1997 was visiting the clock tower face, within the Town Hall in Brisbane. Once we had reached the clock face, I was so excited because it felt like I could see the entire city; though mum didn't feel the same way as me because she has a fear of heights. But a few minutes later it was my turn to feel scared when I heard just how loud the chimes were, which to most adults and children were not too loud. Even today I have a strong sensitivity to any kind of noise around me.

Despite not generally paying attention to calendars at the age of seven, I did have a good look at one that weekend. It was Saturday June the 14th and I was extremely excited because I counted out how there were 'only' 24 more weeks until my birthday. What made me so excited was that for a short while 24 weeks sounded the same as 24 days. I completely overlooked the fact that I'd be very disappointed if I multiplied 24 by 7, thus realising that it was actually closer to 168 days (in 1997 my birthday fell on a Thursday, not a Saturday).

Though I finally realised something on the car journey home that night. I told my grandmother that a year isn't really a long time, and as it was after 6pm I would never again experience 5pm on that exact same date (the exact same year included). Then nana told me that a year isn't a very long time, and that I should treasure every hour of my life that I live, because it's true that we will never again experience that exact same time and date. We also can not make ourselves younger again or fully correct our past mistakes. Nowadays I'm fully aware that this is unfortunately very true indeed.

Hence the reason for why 1997 moved along very quickly, and then in November of that year I had my third ballet concert (this time with the theme of Peter Pan). Me and my classmates were dressed as mermaids and it was another enjoyable experience. Prior to going out mum took a picture of me and Jessica in our costumes.

Yet I thought it would be funny to stick my tongue out as the camera flashed. Mum didn't notice that until she got the photos developed a couple of weeks later, and she wasn't at all pleased. Taking photos back in the nineties wasn't nearly as simple as it is today.

Once technology can do more and more things, it's almost as if we become lazier from all of the laborious jobs it so effortlessly does. However as technology progresses we aren't as excused as we previously were, and should therefore be able to perform tasks to an even greater level than we could achieve in earlier days.

Nowadays, the latest technology is very welcome in my life, as I require various kinds of assistance with my anxiety and disabilities. Back in 1997 it would be several decades before I could significantly be helped from available technology. Though having lived in both kinds of worlds (with and without technology) I can certainly say from experience that I prefer today's world. In upcoming chapters you will read about how I struggled with many situations that could have easily been helped by having an iPad to ground myself with. Yet even in the days before my favourite digital sandbox game Minecraft and 24/7 streaming apps (available at the time of me writing this, in 2021), I did somehow manage to survive.

CHAPTER NINE

FORMING FRIENDSHIPS WITH PEERS FROM MUTUAL INTERESTS

My birthday of 1997 fell on the same day as our class' end of year break-up party. So when I and the rest of the class turned up with a cake, the teachers received a slight shock to discover that mine was a birthday cake with candles to light. The cake was Minnie and Mickey Mouse themed, and the cream was fresh (meaning that it wasn't mock cream) despite being coloured.

Exactly two weeks later was Christmas Day and when me and Jessica woke up early in the morning we were surprised to see our new inflatable pool. In truth the water was only a foot and a half deep. But we thoroughly enjoyed cooling down on a hot summer's day by swimming in it, with our hands and feet crawling along the bottom.

Continuing on into Grade Three brings along some more gradual changes. I didn't do as much screaming and crying at school anymore, even though social awkwardness was definitely still present (as it is to this day). Unlike the previous two years however, I didn't fully withdraw myself from my peers.

At the beginning of the year our school had a competition where children had to dress up as any fictional character. I chose Ariel from The Little Mermaid, and wore my mermaid costume (from the previous ballet concert I had) with red coloured hairspray. For that impersonation I ended up winning second place, and won a few dollars to spend on sweets from the canteen.

A few months later, I developed a certain interest, that (for the first time) wasn't unexpected for a child my age.

As was the case with most young girls in 1998 I was a huge fan of the Spice Girls, and boasted a collection of all five of the dolls. This interest made me willing to socialise with my peers a little bit more. So many girls at school would put on impersonating concerts during recess breaks singing Spice Girls songs.

That year my grandparents went to the UK for a few weeks to see our family there. Me and Jessica couldn't go, yet nana told us that she would bring us home a complete set of the Spice Dolls. When they returned home we were thrilled to bits and very thankful. In addition to the Spice Dolls we were also given heaps of candy, including some featuring Jetsons characters.

However there was a very exciting event at one of our local shopping centres while our grandparents were away, which I enjoyed a lot. One of my favourite shows on TV, the quiz show Sale of the Century had travelled up to Queensland. They held a quiz show onstage for members of the public to be contestants and win prizes. Unfortunately to compete there was a minimum age requirement of 16. Yet the hosts of the show still brought me onstage, and gave me some questions more suitable for an 8–12 year old child to answer in front of everyone. The geography questions were of course my favourite kind!

While we're on the topic of geography, our class at school also participated in a very fun exchange program with a class of the same age group in Hong Kong. We shared different kinds of lessons with each other and knowledge about our own places of the world via email, which at that time was rather new technology. There was another very interesting activity that we did. The kids in our class took it in turns to take a giant toy panda home with us for the night, and if we were well behaved it would be for a whole weekend, for those like myself who were lucky enough to take the panda home on a Friday.

Whereas we had sent the class in Hong Kong a giant plush koala for the kids there to do the same as we did. Each class had to write a short piece about what our plush toy did in our homes. Afterward we got to learn about the similarities and differences about childhood in different parts of the world.

With all of those memorable events of 1998 (of which you have just read about in this chapter), I can positively say that it was one of my happiest childhood years! Then, once November came along, there was another dance concert (this time with the theme of The Nutcracker), and I was dressed as a red and gold toy soldier. However that year me and Jessica decided to try out tap dancing instead of ballet for a change. I preferred tap dancing to ballet as there was more stress relieving action involved, and due to my autism I enjoy counting and making physical actions to rhythm.

However, I perhaps needed to persist with this new activity for a couple more years, until the novelty of it wore off.

CHAPTER TEN

NIGHTTIME TERRORS

When my 9th birthday came around in December, 1998 it took me a long time to get to sleep due to my intense excitement. However I did finally fall asleep and woke up to receive a toy stable (the size of a dollhouse) which included a few plastic horses. My grandparents came to visit me at lunchtime, and then we spent the rest of the afternoon swimming and relaxing at South Bank in Brisbane.

On Christmas Day (a fortnight later) the presents I received were several Skydancers (popular spinning toy dolls in the 1990s), a Sale of the Century and Wheel of Fortune board game, a dinosaur hand puppet and several inflatable pool toys to use at our grandparents' house or at South Bank. I was also given a few 200 piece Disney jigsaw puzzles of which I enjoyed putting together for most of the day.

Yet while I was putting the jigsaws together I experienced a feeling of intense sadness, as my mind was going through thoughts as I was working on the puzzles. I got a realisation that Christmas of 1998 (which I had been looking forward to for almost a whole year) would never happen again. By lunchtime, half of that Christmas was already wiped away into the past, permanently. It had been such an enjoyable time, though it would never again be experienced and would become a mere memory. Admittedly this made me cry privately to myself. Even at the age of nine I was too embarrassed to reveal this to anybody. But I couldn't help feeling so upset because the transition of enjoyable times into intangible memories is just so sad.

My next year of school (Grade Four) was a significant time for me, mainly because I had such a nice teacher who helped me along.

However, during that year I still dreaded recess due to a combination of bullying and having poor social skills. Thus, I was only getting an hour or two of sleep each night as a result of the stress.

CHAPTER TEN

Falling asleep became an obsession, and wanting to fall asleep when we are not able to makes insomnia worse. There had always been nights when I found it difficult to fall asleep. Though 1999 was the first year when I had so many sleepless nights that I had a bout of insomnia.

At that time (and still to this day) I feared seeing the sun coming up before I had any sleep at all since bedtime. The whole concept of that happening was frightening to me because I viewed the normal procedure as being a sequence of going to bed, falling asleep and then waking up in the morning. Even when I think of any of those steps being missed it's terrifying for me, because it feels so unnatural and unsafe. I strongly feel that any action that it not biologically supposed to happen to us is not recommended, and therefore not proven to be 100% safe.

During that time I was also having nightmares whenever I did manage to fall asleep (and we usually dream whilst we are in lighter sleep). Those nightmares were being fed to me by a person in my waking life describing the process of damnation to me in horrific detail, and how I would end up burning in hell after I died. Thus I was having constant nightmares involving this person's face growing devil horns, and sinking into a burning grave. As he was sinking he would be sniggering at me, and saying (in a childlike whining tone) "Where's Becky? I want Becky". In my waking life this person would too snigger at me like that, and would also use that same childish tone while he was bullying me. Though by merely adding devil horns to his actual face, words, actions and character, he appeared to be so much scarier than he was in the real world.

This stage of my life wasn't only a pain for me. Is was an absolute nightmare for the rest of the family, and (it would be wrong for me not to say this here) the whole neighbourhood too. As a result of being terrified to see the clock quickly winding towards sunrise, I would scream at the top of my voice in the middle of the night. In absolute honesty I did not do this with the intention of keeping everyone else awake. The truth was that I would see that it was 3am, knew that I had to get up to go to school in a mere three hours, and thus I would have an uncontrollable meltdown.

In the time span from my birth to the present day I have experienced an enormous number of meltdowns, and I must admit too that I haven't escaped three decades of my life without having at least a few dozen immature temper tantrums (especially given that this includes my infant and toddler years). Yet from experiencing episodes of both, I am now able to see a very clear difference between the two.

Especially in my earlier years of childhood (prior to school age) I would have a temper tantrum in a fully conscious and controlled manner, for the purpose of either getting something I wanted, or to make myself heard to receive sympathy. There is even emotional manipulation and blackmail involved in that as well. Children are certainly not sweet and innocent *all* of the time; there may be some extremely rare exceptions, but I was not one of them.

Though in the case of a meltdown it's done in a much less organised and a very uncontrolled manner. It begins by experiencing a situation which brings about strong feelings (such as fear, excitement, anger or sadness) which are difficult for me to understand the meaning or cause of. From there, the inability for me to be able to cope with such a strong emotion (either negative or positive) is what causes the outburst itself. This is the reason why it is difficult at first for me or my family to pinpoint what exactly it was that brought about the meltdown, as the cause was simply an inability to handle an emotion itself.

It's very challenging for me to describe the exact feeling of a meltdown in words. Yet I'll attempt this by saying that it feels as if those misunderstood emotions are electrified to around 1000 volts, and my heart rate increases dramatically. This has usually been to around 225bpm, yet during a very intense meltdown it was once measured to be at 317bpm (which is extremely dangerous).

As a result of that, both my mind and body regress to the basic coping method of yelling, screaming and thrashing around on the floor. To the present day I am gradually improving, as throughout the years this has been one of the primary focuses of my continued therapy. It's essential for me to control my extreme moments of anxiety with mindfulness (by doing Minecraft, using fidget spinners and doing mindfulness colouring), instead of falling back towards the basic, immature and more primitive method of having a meltdown.

In Grade Four I had my first school camp, and nighttime was of course a disaster. In fact I experienced a fair bit of bullying for a while in regards to the meltdowns I had in front of my whole school grade. Though just as is the case with all meltdowns, it doesn't matter where I am or who is in front of me. If they occur, I simply cannot stop myself regardless of who is present and how embarrassed I feel.

Something else that I didn't fancy about my first camp was that the environment was very different to how it was at home. I must add here that I did enjoy the beautiful hinterland scenery of waterfalls, trekking through rainforests and seeing a few glow-worms in a cave for the first time. Being in that peaceful environment calmed me immensely. Yet the campsite itself was a different story.

I had never camped before, and camping does take some getting used to. We slept in simple bunkbeds in cabins where there were holes in the whitewashed brick walls. There was also the occasional scribble or two on the walls, where kids had done some cheeky drawings with a few swear words. However, eating the food which was provided there was perhaps the most difficult thing for me.

On our first day we used the dining room to learn some simple dancing exercises. I knew that I would enjoy this, as dancing along to polkas and jigs is a good way for me to zone out. But I was horrified at the sight of the kitchen as we walked past it. I thought that it looked old, extremely ugly and very dirty. Nowadays I'm fully aware that many campsite and industrial kitchens look like that. But at nine years old I thought differently. I couldn't see how such an old fashioned fridge (which was hardly more advanced than an icebox) would keep the food fresh. I also couldn't see how an antiquated stove and utensils would be able to cook the bacteria out of the food. There were many oil splashes and soup stains all over the place too.

Every time we ate a meal that had been cooked or prepared in that kitchen I felt like vomiting. Visual memories of the kitchen made the food taste disgusting. So I decided in a childish way that I wouldn't eat until I was back at home. But a girl at my table noticed that I had made this decision and 'dobbed me in' for it.

A teacher then said that I was being a baby and they were going to make sure that I finished my meals. So I made sure I picked food that I knew I couldn't get food poisoning from. Unfortunately this too was noticed, and I got told to eat food that would fill me up. Therefore I was given a large piece of lasagne, which was full of meat and dairy. There was no way I could finish it on time, so like an immature child I threw it into the food scraps bin when the teachers weren't looking. I felt too embarrassed to tell anyone that I wasn't eating due to fears of germs and food poisoning. Feeling hungry was much easier than feeling scared was. Thus overall, my first school camp wasn't a great success, unfortunately.

But on a much happier note, the year 1999 was the time when I got introduced to the *Harry Potter* series, which have remained to be such a huge part of my life.

My teacher (who also looked after me during that previous camp) knew that I despised recess and that I liked to sit alone for most of the time. So she mentioned to my mother that she had come across a new book series. Mum was told that it's about a boy who feels lonely and different, until he discovers that he's a wizard, and is then sent to a magical school called Hogwarts.

I'd never heard of the *Harry Potter* series at that time and I had never taken to fiction books previously. My preferences were still atlases and encyclopaedias. Therefore initially I didn't think I would enjoy the *Harry Potter* books. However after being constantly asked, I finally accepted my teacher's suggestion of reading her copy of *Harry Potter and the Philosopher's Stone* during recess break.

Incredibly, it didn't take long for me to like the book enough to buy a copy for myself! From that moment on I've read all of the books and watched all of the movies over and over. I've also learned to recite the *Harry Potter* books word by word. So you'll hear a lot more about *Harry Potter* throughout the rest of my own book.

CHAPTER ELEVEN

MY FIRST EXPERIENCE OF TRAVELLING OVERSEAS

Moving on to Grade Five, I can say too that the year 2000 was one of my most eventful years. The year did of course begin with a *massive* New Year's Eve celebration. We had a street party and we filled up an inflatable swimming pool in our front garden (New Year falls in Summer in the Southern Hemisphere). We had a heap of neon glow sticks as usual, and party accessories with the number 2000 written all over them.

At the age of ten I was able to *mostly* acknowledge the significance of the event (the beginning of a new year, a new decade, a new century and a new millennium in combination). However, I regret not being *quite* old enough to be fully motivated to stay up until midnight without constantly dozing off. I needed to stay clear of the numerous fireworks that were going off as well, because the noise of them terrified me.

But all in all, I did have a very enjoyable night where I got to socialise with other children in the neighbourhood, and the celebrations seemed to have lasted throughout the remainder of January.

Once I returned to school I was happy that I got the same teacher as I had the previous year. That was also the time when I had my first experience of being elected as a Class Captain. Each year every school kid wanted that position as they would get to wear a badge and would be given certain privileges that other students didn't have.

Even so there was a hiccup when another teacher unexpectedly quit their job. This meant that all of the school's Grade 5 classes had to get reshuffled around, as they said that it was impossible to employ someone else to replace the initial teacher's post. The school principal even visited our class to say that ours was the class which would be changed the most! I was very worried about that because I had a close relationship with my teacher and I would also lose the position of being a class leader (prior to even getting a badge to keep). Though I was really thankful when it turned out that I got to remain in the same class.

In April of that year I had my second school camp. This time, having experienced a school camp previously it wasn't quite as difficult for me. While we were up on the Sunshine Coast we did some fishing, canoeing and we got to spend a lot of time at the beach. On our first day at the beach I was intrigued by the sight of a huge cargo ship out at sea. Then on our second day something hilarious had happened. The lifeguards were suddenly yelling at all of us kids from across the beach, telling us to stay out of the water because there was a shark. From my viewpoint it was quite amusing as everyone was yelling and screaming at this single fin, that was just drifting peacefully along the water. It's incredible how such dangerous things can have the appearance of being so subtle, at first glance.

This time eating at the campsite wasn't a problem for me. I had grown familiar with the fact that campsite facilities aren't quite as nice as everyday facilities. I also met the people who would be cooking the food and they appeared to be trustworthy. Due to the difficulties I had on my previous camp the teachers looked after me more so the second time. Me and a fellow student (who had anxiety disorders like myself) got a suite instead of a cabin, which even had a bathroom and laundry attached. My insomnia and nighttime meltdowns had by then subsided, for the meantime.

As is the case with most disabilities, my autism and OCD magnifies whenever I'm under stress. On my Grade Four camp the screaming at night was due to my autism, and my fear of bacteria in the food was due to my Obsessive Compulsive Disorder. However throughout the year 2000, when I was in Grade Five I wasn't experiencing an excessive amount of stress.

In September of that year I went on another school trip, this time to the North Island of New Zealand. That became the best school camp that I had ever had! The purpose of this two week long camp was for us to learn about the Maori culture.

Earlier that year Jessica and I were half excited about the possibility of our New Zealand trip, and half disappointed because there was (initially) a strong probability that we wouldn't be able to go. Though, once it was certain that we would be going overseas we were busy at work raising money for the trip.

It was a lot of work, but all for a good purpose. Our extracurricular class raised money by washing cars, delivering phone books to houses and doing market stalls. So much work was done in a short space of time, which is a lot for a group of children (some as young as five years old), but the good news was that we successfully got there in the end!

Our flight from Brisbane to Auckland was on September the 12th of that year. At the time I was excited and also very nervous. We had never been away from mum for two whole weeks. We also had no idea what being on an aeroplane would be like, and our mind had of course been poisoned by some people telling us about plane crashes. As well, we had never been overseas beforehand. Once we entered customs it made us sad to see mum waving us off and crying. But she was crying because she was happy, more so than sad. Mum definitely wasn't the only parent acting that way.

Once we entered the aircraft it looked far more comfortable than I expected it to be. The three hour flight was smooth with very little turbulence. Jessica and I brought some toys to keep us entertained (given to us by our mother). Mine was a toy much like an etch-a-sketch, except that it featured a face on which I could draw hair with a magnetic pen and iron fillings. Though I never ended up playing with that, as I was far more interested in watching the map showing our flight progress. Whenever I see any kind of map it never fails to keep me entertained for hours. We also had a delicious dinner and lots of chocolate treats for dessert.

In September, New Zealand is two hours ahead of us. As it was midnight in Auckland we arrived at the airport when it was very quiet. All of us kids were excited about being in another country, while the airport staff were almost falling asleep at their desks.

This was the very first time I had flown anywhere, and therefore customs and border security were extremely new to me (in fact those experiences do still give me extreme anxiety to this day). On that night I had a drink bottle filled with water which I had been given with my dinner during the flight. While I walked through the sensor the alarm went off and all of the other children were staring at me. The woman who oversaw the matter certainly wasn't the warmest person I've come across while going through customs. She didn't speak to me in a tone that one would normally use for a child of ten. Her cold words were "There appears to be something suspicious in your bag. We'll thoroughly search you, and then we will deal with you accordingly".

While I was being searched I burst into tears. Yet once I was given the all clear, there was no apology or any kind of empathy from her. The woman clearly couldn't care less that I was a child with severe anxiety, in addition to having other developmental disabilities which made me even younger psychologically. It was true that I was tall for my age and experienced a severe bout of acne very early. Yet that doesn't change the actual age of a child.

Anyhow, I quickly recovered from that issue when I left the airport and saw another country (in person and not by a photo in a book) for the first time in my life. New Zealand is such a different place, in comparison to Brisbane geologically. Here at home there are gumtrees everywhere we look. Yet in New Zealand you see snowcapped mountains wherever you look. It was also very cold outside of the airport.

We then boarded a bus to take us down to Waitara (near New Plymouth). It was a very long ride and a few movies were played on the way down there. Some children watched Mr. Bean, while others including myself (even though I find Mr. Bean hilarious) just watched mountain after mountain pass the windows.

In the peace and silence of the night, the sight of those dark mountains truly did seem to tell us a deep story as old as the land itself. Strangely, no spoken words were needed for us to be entertained by this.

There were some children who even voiced that all of the dark and solemn looking trees standing countlessly in the countryside (undisturbed by any urban building), looked just like ancient people and warriors greeting us to the land. There has never been another moment in my life when I was told such a rich story without any verbal or written information. Rather than being eerie, it was in fact very magical. All of the other children and teachers shared that same viewpoint.

Hardly anyone slept that night and at dawn we finally stopped at a small inn next to a beach with black volcanic sand. The air was very cold and I could literally taste the frost in my mouth every time I breathed it in. Luckily the inn where we ate breakfast at was heated nicely, and I had a meal containing whitebait (a traditional New Zealand fish).

Afterward we visited a local school who welcomed us greatly. All of us guest children were divided up into groups, and then we attended different classes with the school's children for that day. The classrooms looked very different from our own. In this small town of New Zealand the school desks were made of sturdy wood where the top could be pulled up, in order to take out the stationary stored within them. Our own school desks merely had a plastic 'tidy-tray' to store our books and pencils in, which just slid in and out, and sometimes even crashed onto the floor with too much weight. The class we visited also had composite grades, which were Fourth Grade and Ninth Grade together. All of us guests were given a free lunch and even a piece of chocolate cake for an afternoon dessert.

Later on that day we travelled to the Marae where we would be spending the night. We were very privileged to have been invited by local Maori communities to sleep in and eat at these splendid places all throughout our trip. It was natural for us children to be feeling homesick (especially those of us who's parents didn't come along). Yet the sight of those beautiful carved pillars and the paintings of local myths and legends took away all thoughts of wanting to be back at home. If only the Pixar film *Moana* had been released a couple of decades earlier! But there was a town called *Moana* that we visited during our trip. I often wonder if the film was named after that beautiful place.

Us children even got to see some natural snow for the first time in our life. We took a bus to the top of Mt. Ruapehu, almost reaching the massive caldera that loomed overhead. Then we all had much fun playing in the slushy snow and tobogganing down the hills. Something else that we got to see while we were away from home were the hot springs of Rotorua. The sight of the park we visited, with its steam and bubbling mud, was so fantastic that it enabled us to tolerate the strong smell of sulphur.

We ended our trip back in Auckland and got to have a good look around the city. Compared to most other cities and towns in New Zealand, Auckland is a big place! Auckland reminds me very much of my hometown in quite a number of ways. We went to the city museum and attended a workshop about the Maori culture, then afterward we watched an insightful performance.

Finally and sadly, the moment came when it was time for us to return home. On this occasion my experience while going through customs was in stark contrast to how it was at the beginning of the trip. The woman checking my bags was a lovely person. She spoke to me very kindly and told me not to worry about the occasional staff members who are rude. Me and my teachers were also told that I should never have been treated so badly upon my arrival, and I was asked to give a description of the officer who did so.

The moral of this story was for me to know that despite there being occasional people who are unpleasant to me in life, there are many more who acknowledge how wrong it is for a person to be treated so unkindly. Therefore I needed to develop more trust in the people of the world and to know that not everyone has intentions of harming me. Today I have come to realise that those previous feelings I would experience were a result of my Post Traumatic Stress Disorder. The therapy I was receiving was a godsend for that.

Once I had learned this important life lesson, I was able to trust people enough to make some more friends a few months afterward, in the following school year.

CHAPTER TWELVE

NOW I ACTUALLY WANT TO SPEND MORE TIME WITH MY FRIENDS THAN DOING MY SCHOOLWORK

Grade Six was a year that also rolled along fantastically, and not because of any school trips. Instead, it was because I made a group of friends who I would talk to constantly, and we would even see each other at places outside of school. Beforehand there were fellow students who I acquainted myself with and who were very kind to me. Yet the case was different with Elanah, Lauren and Monica because there wasn't a day during school or the weekends/holidays when I didn't see or hear from them.

There were even many occasions when I preferred socialising with them, rather than reading my books and studying. That's a very unusual, yet by all means positive feeling for me.

However on a much bleaker note, throughout that year I was suffering from repeated boils, as a result of a staphylococcus infection which I had caught the previous year. Boils are the most painful thing I have experienced as yet. They're highly contagious, so I was getting about three boils at a time, and new ones would appear as soon as each healed. I've experienced boils on every part of my body and I'd have to say that the inner thigh area is the most painful. Whenever I'd get a boil there it was agony to walk, sit down, stand up or move my leg at all (as the whole leg became purple and swollen).

Lancing, dressing, and in particular bursting the boil made me scream uncontrollably. They said that there was nothing which could be done to treat the infection; so I would have to wait a long time for the virus to come out of my system. That ended up taking two years, which was both an emotional and physical pain.

Due to getting continuous boils I had to take a lot of time off dancing. By then I had a good try of ballet and tap dancing. While I had taken time away from that I had consequently realised that dancing wasn't really my kind of thing. My hand-eye coordination wasn't too good, and as I was progressing into the higher levels this was becoming more and more necessary. So that year was when dancing became an activity of the past for me.

However I cannot close this year off without mentioning the fabulous *Harry Potter* themed birthday I had when I turned twelve. There was a moment in July of that year when I asked Mum if I could have my bedroom painted like Hogwarts castle. Even so, I was half expecting that my mum would say no, due to the amount of work and money that would be involved in that.

However, I was ecstatic when I got told that she *could* do that, but to bear in mind that I wouldn't be able to have as many other presents to open on that day. Mum began painting the room during the first week of December, and for a whole week I wasn't allowed in there and had to sleep on the floor of Jessica's room. Though on the morning of my birthday I was in awe as I stepped into my bedroom, that looked just like the Hogwarts I imagined to exist in the *Harry Potter* books.

Then after we had breakfast, Mum took me, Elanah and Monica to see the film of *Harry Potter and the Philosopher's Stone*, and it was fantastic. Later on in the day, many more guests came along for a dinner of pizzas at our house. We couldn't have been happier about the number of people who came, knowing that this *Harry Potter* themed birthday meant the absolute world to me.

My interest in the *Harry Potter* series stayed with me for a very long time. Indeed if the character himself didn't wear glasses, it would have made my diagnosis of myopia (short-sightedness) the following year far more challenging.

CHAPTER THIRTEEN

MY LIFE IS CHANGING WHETHER I WANT IT TO OR NOT

Grade Seven was when I truly began to fall behind and struggle with my schoolwork. Primary school is much more structured and involves less hypothetical assessments (in both exams and assignments).

During the first half of our twelve year school life we can receive good marks and be positively praised by teachers, merely by listing all of the world's capital cities, acing spelling tests, rote learning information and so forth.

From that, many teachers are given a false impression that primary school students like I myself was, will have no difficulties with schooling and their future careers. Yet there comes a time half way through our years at school when simply knowing the 'black and white' answers to everything is purely and simply not good enough anymore. More rather, it reaches a point when we must explain by using hundreds of words the reasons for 'why' those are indeed the answers, whenever we are given assessments. That I struggle with enormously. Even in social conversations I have a lot of difficulty when I have to turn a factual sentence of ten words, into a conversation of five hundred words.

In Grade Seven I was not coping well with school at all. I didn't act out, though I wasn't able to keep up with various assessments that had different due dates. The way my mind operates is that I must be given single tasks with a due date and time set. Once I've completed a task, that's when I'll begin work on the next, and the sequence continues.

School assignments however aren't given to us in that way. While we're working on one assignment, we're often unexpectedly given another two or more by different classes to work on simultaneously.

To make matters even more confusing, they're never due on the same date!

In addition to that I was also getting bullied by a girl who was two grades below me. She didn't seem to care that I had friends sitting with me and teachers nearby, as she was very glad to bully and physically assault me, regardless of who was present. This girl would painfully punch me, and give me derogative names due to the fact that I was different. She would too (rather cruelly) invite her friends along. This wasn't for the purpose of them supporting her, but so that they could get a laugh at my reactions as she was hurting me. The school were informed about those incidents, and they helped in the best way that they could.

Yet at least it was then not a long time until I moved on to a secondary school which she didn't attend. Her name has not been given here, as I did end up discovering in the years afterward that she became a much nicer person as she matured into adulthood. There was even a moment when she willingly approached me with a sincere apology a few years later.

As well as being bullied by that girl, there was an afternoon in July of 2002 when some kids were walking past our house, on their way home from school. They didn't come to our door but were talking to each other loudly as they walked by.

While I was cuddling our new kitten (Lilly-Rose), the words which initially caught my attention were "You know this house don't you? It's where that crazy freak, Rebecca Sharrock lives". I knew that they were talking about me because 'Sharrock' was not a common surname. Then they went on to say "Apparently, it's supposed to be a 'nuthouse', and they never wash themselves. That's why her face is covered with eczema".

After hearing this, Jessica informed us that a few of her classmates had asked whether our house really was infested by dirt and rats. They also told Jessica that they couldn't hang around with her, because their parents had warned them about us 'being a bad influence' on them.

All of that made me very upset and I burst into tears. Mum was hurt and infuriated as well.

In addition to those three issues I mentioned above, I was given a lot of criticism about my unusually early and severe acne. My skin has always been prone to outbreaks of boils and acne (during times of extreme stress), which made my skin from Grades 4–7 terrible. I'd have to use pharmaceutical soaps and medication specifically made for severe cases of acne. To this day I'm still allergic to any kind of soap, apart from QV wash which I get from our local pharmacy. Even the fluoride which is added to tap water gives me severe reactions.

For me, breakouts of acne haven't just been confined to my preteen and teenage years. It is indeed a lifelong ailment which I get with my type of skin. Today I still do get intense outbreaks of acne in summer and/or whenever I'm stressed. It was the exact same too when I was as young as five years old.

The year 2002 was when I started having to wear glasses as well. There was a day when I was copying down something from the blackboard, and I realised that it was too blurry for me to read. Mum who wears glasses herself knew the right optician to take me to and we found out that I had myopia (or short sightedness). I was partially upset because I could no longer do things like watching television while falling asleep, or seeing the time from the other end of my room as soon as I woke up. Glasses also get water droplets on them in the rain, and they have to be cleaned at least four times a day.

Yet it was a blessing that I liked the *Harry Potter* series so much, because the character Harry himself is short sighted and wears glasses just like me.

Also, while we are on the topic of *Harry Potter*, in November of that year mum took me and my friends out again to see the film *Harry Potter and the Chamber of Secrets*. While we were there we had chocolate frogs, liquorice wands and Bertie Botts beans to munch on. In 2002 those edible treats were available, even though they were different from those of today.

Of course, Grade Seven was the year we graduated from primary school in the state of Queensland a couple of decades ago. My graduation day was an extremely enjoyable event, and much better than I could ever have anticipated! Certain students won trophies for different kinds of achievements, and me and my three best friends all won a trophy (mine was in the area of academics)!

Afterwards me, my friends and classmates enjoyed pizzas that the school provided for us all, in addition to a celebration disco. Yet I didn't participate in much dancing, nor did I grab second and third servings of pizza. Instead me and my friends did our socialising outside in a courtyard. Most of what we were talking about was how much we enjoyed our time together, in a school of which we would no longer be pupils at in a mere few days from then.

CHAPTER FOURTEEN

ADJUSTING TO A NEW SCHOOL WITH NEW FRIENDSHIPS TO MAKE

The following year I began Grade Eight at Calamvale Community College. It was a brand new school that had opened close to where I live. Despite Calamvale being a public school, it ran very differently from others of it's kind. Our lessons weren't based on the set curriculum that state schools were usually run by. In fact Calamvale was a pilot school to figure out the best ways of educating the children of the future (even if it was by trial and error at occasional times). As a result of this we would have countless visitors from universities and other schools, who would come to our classes to observe how everything worked out.

Calamvale Community College was so named because it is a kindergarten, primary school and high school all combined as one. Junior school was years 1–6 (divided into lower and upper), middle school was years 7–9 and senior school was years 10–12 (though in 2003 the school only went up to Grade 9). Each sub school had it's own canteen, classrooms and facilities. The only places that the whole school shared were the library and the main administration building. Due to the large number of students, each sub school arrived and departed from the campus at different times. I was in middle school then. So we started our school day at 8:30am and finished at 2:30pm.

Beginning high school wasn't quite as scary for me as my experience of beginning Grade One. It was of course a different campus, but after seven years of previous schooling I did have an inkling of what it was all about. As an autistic person the social issues of starting at a new school weren't a cause of concern for me. Being in the company of peers on our first day of school isn't crucially important for many autistic children.

We generally don't mind sitting alone and entertaining ourselves by our own thoughts.

I did indeed have friends, but something that I'm very thankful for is that I didn't walk through the school gates feeling pressured to make friends. Those lovely peers of mine simply approached me, I got to know them well, and thanks to social media I haven't lost contact with them.

My first term (January-March) was an interesting experience. The major project was called 'Back To The Future' and yes, we did get to watch the film of the same name in class. Yet our main project was for us to imagine how ourselves and the world would change in decades to come.

The concept of the whole term was rather confusing for me, due to my difficulties with understanding what the seemingly undefined moments of time were (despite the future being certain it's still unknown of in the present time). In other words I found it extremely challenging to think of myself as an older person in the future. That had nothing to do with worries about ageing. Instead, it was a feeling of uncertainty when it came to imagining myself and my life experiences in a time which I had not yet experienced. When it came to the past (even from much younger ages), it was different because I had memories of my psychological self from those times.

Despite the fact that my confusion didn't completely disappear when it came to being a different person from an unknown time, it was very helpful to grasp an understanding that my present self is what influences my future self. A less complex way of saying this is that it's psychologically very helpful to remind myself of the words "just imagine how much your future self will thank you by putting in the effort, being strong and doing this work now, to make things easier for you in her/my time". Also, it brings a smile to my face when I eventually *become* that future self and *remember* the moment when I told myself the words mentioned above. That particular concept has had a huge impact on my life today, and I'll bring that up again in a later chapter.

Aside from that there was also a lot happening in the media, and all of that did work it's way into our lessons and conversations amongst the other students. In February of 2003 the space shuttle (Columbia) disaster covered the media. All astronauts on board tragically died when their shuttle disintegrated during re-entering the Earth's atmosphere. It was being compared to the Challenger disaster of 1986. Though I don't of course have any memories of that particular disaster as it happened three years before I even existed.

In early March I had my next dramatic injury after the time when I cut my eyebrow open as a three year old. One of my best friends Elanah lived in a house which was walking distance from ours. So on a Sunday morning I rode my scooter to her house. While I was there we watched the DVD I had brought along, which was a thriller movie.

At 4pm Elanah and I decided that it was time to return to my own house (Elanah decided to accompany me there). She took her bicycle and I rode on my early 2000s metal scooter. Unfortunately the road turning onto our house faces directly west, so you could just imagine the problems that would cause in the late afternoon. The sun was directly in my eyes and it got to a point where I couldn't see a thing.

Yet as I was about to get off the scooter and walk along the footpath (according to our law it is illegal to ride anything with wheels on a footpath), I very unluckily hit this tiny pebble. An air-filled tyre would simply ride over it. But a vehicle with solid rubber wheels and very little suspension is a different story. When I hit the stone my scooter flung onto the footpath and escaped damage. I however fell straight down onto the side of the road and copped a fair few grazes.

But it didn't stop there. Just as I thought 'it's only a few grazes' my mouth smashed into the ground with so much force that it shattered my front teeth!

From the time I walked home to the time I went to bed I was screaming. Pretty much anyone can imagine why a thirteen year old girl would do so. It had nothing whatsoever to do with the pain I was in. Whenever I smiled into a mirror, all I saw were jagged roughly cut 'rocks', which were all that remained of my front teeth. As it was a Sunday all dentists were closed. So I spent the night with smashed teeth, and much of the next day being unable to speak discernibly.

First thing next morning Mum took me to the dental hospital. It wasn't a 'first in best dressed' service there. Instead everyone was given a number at the door which varied anywhere from 1 to over 100. We were (very luckily) given the number 5. As we walked up to the service desk it was obvious by the look of my bruises, grazes and broken teeth that I was the patient who needed to be attended to. Yet the woman's immediate question was about how old I was, because we then found out that they didn't treat anyone under the age of sixteen. So by law they couldn't treat me there, and they gave us the contact details of a paediatric dentist.

After I was sent home, I had a tin of Heinz tomato soup for lunch while Mum was on the phone to the dentist. At that time the only places local to us that treated children's teeth were in mobile vans at schools. Once I had finished my soup mum took me to the nearest dental van to my school.

The dentist and nurse who treated me were lovely. They greeted me with a smile and asked straight away about whether it was a scooter or a bike. I was assured that I wasn't the only person it had happened to, and that once they'd reconstructed my teeth (for no charge as I was a minor) hardly anyone would notice.

The material used to reconstruct my teeth was composite resin, which is the exact same material currently used for dental fillings. A definite advantage of the teeth already being broken was that no drilling was needed. Afterward they looked as good as new, and I couldn't even tell that they'd been broken, unless I looked very closely and saw the line connecting the caps to the teeth.

However we were still told that caps aren't quite as strong as genuine teeth and do need to get replaced every now and again. We were also told that a knock as severe as the one I had experienced *could* kill the nerve in the tooth itself (that's when it turns black). Yet I am very fortunate that this did not end up happening to me, and those caps have lasted to the present day.

A mere two months later, Mum and Jessica were in a different situation. They had gone out on a wet Thursday evening to do the weekly grocery shopping. Due to the large amount of homework that I had to complete for school (and also due to the fact that I was then older), I was allowed to stay at home while the other two went out. I had remained at home by myself three times beforehand and enjoyed the novelty back then.

Maybe it was to do with the miserable weather that night, I'm not too sure. However on that particular occasion I felt the intense sensation of being alone (at night) for the very first time. While mum was out a friend of hers called, and when I answered the phone with "Hi, it's Becky. Mum isn't home right now but you can call back in a couple of hours", I was told to never give my name out in a phone call and say that I was alone at nighttime. This made the silence feel even deeper, and every mechanical clock in the house ticked louder. It was a very eerie feeling. As a result of that I was unable to concentrate on my schoolwork.

At around 7:30pm the phone rang again, and all I could hear were sirens and my mother's voice in very poor reception. The phone then cut out, and I was in such a worried state that I couldn't do any more of my homework. Twenty minutes later another family friend came to the door and informed me that Mum and Jessica had just been in a car crash. She said that she would drive me to the hospital to meet them. This made me very concerned, and I immediately asked if they were okay. She then assured me that their injuries were only minor.

When we met up with them we heard all the details about the crash. Mum and Jessica were filtering into a lane when a car hit them from behind. They were then knocked into the middle of the busy road, and got hit again at 80kph from the side of the car. Mum's glasses had also flung off in the crash and her eyesight's so bad that she's unable to see anything without them.

The car ended up getting written off due to extensive damage. So another family friend (Tania) drove me and Jessica to and from school for a week. This gave us an opportunity to have nightly sleepovers for a whole week at her house, and we were thrilled about this as Tania's daughter Elanah is one of my closest friends. While we were there we had so much fun.

Throughout that year Jessica and I would accompany Elanah on a road trip down to the Gold Coast to pick up her two younger half sisters for regular visits. We'd always collect them from their dad by the sea shore. In July it was obviously far too cold for us to swim (July falls in Winter in the Southern Hemisphere). But swimming happens to be a beach activity that I find boring and less appealing. What I liked best was hiking up to the edge of the cliff and looking at the raging waves below, while feeling the fresh breeze against my face. It looked very much like a scene in the film *Harry Potter and the Halfblood Prince* where Harry and Dumbledore are stood atop a cliff by the seashore, about to enter the cave where Lord Voldemort's fake horcrux was hidden. However that film wasn't yet released in 2003, and nor was the book it was based upon.

Virtually every weekend of that year we would visit Warner Brothers Movie World with Elanah. This was because we had yearly passes and liked *Harry Potter* so much. Warner Brothers Movie World is our small local version of the Universal Parks in places like Hollywood and Orlando (those examples were used as I have since visited and enjoyed both of those places). Unfortunately our local park isn't big enough to have individual sub-parks such as Harry Potter World. But much *Harry Potter* merchandise was sold throughout, which was great as there weren't any pop culture stores such as Zing (similar to Hot Topic) local to us back then.

All of those things mentioned just above virtually defined my entire life outside of school that year. But I did still get to experience some very interesting events within school as well.

At the end of September our class held a conference at the University of Queensland which was about genetic engineering. This was also the first time when I realised that I had a liking of public speaking. My teachers knew me to be a quiet and seemingly shy student, so they were slightly hesitant about getting me to do a speech.

Though while I was up on stage I wasn't scared at all, and I did in fact really enjoy myself! I too had to fill in for another student's talk due to her being unable to do so. Once the conference had ended all of my teachers were both surprised and very impressed by my work that day!

Discovering how much I enjoyed public speaking was the very first step towards me realising the career which I wanted to do as an adult. I'm now a professional speaker who delivers work through speeches, public talks, media interviews and writing. This was an important milestone for me, as previously I had never been able to pinpoint (in any way) the career I wanted to have once I had left school.

As we moved into November our pet cat Lilly-Rose had her first litter of kittens in the early hours of the morning, and Mum woke me and Jessica up to watch her give birth to them. Unluckily for mum the cat was on her bed the whole time, which sure did make a mess and a half to clean up afterward! Jessica and I decided to stay awake for the rest of the night to spend time with the kittens. It was 4am anyway, and we had to start getting ready for school only an hour afterward.

That day was Tuesday November the 3rd, and it was also Melbourne Cup Day. For us in Queensland it is not a public holiday, even though we did always watch the horserace in the classroom at 2pm our time (unlike the rest of the Australian east coast, Queensland doesn't have daylight savings). Yet on that particular day the teachers had a surprise for us. Instead of the usual lessons, we did a heap of activities relating to the Melbourne Cup. We made hats, learned about the history of the great race, and (to the delight of many of the teenage students) were taught how to fill out a TAB ticket and put a bet on which horse we thought might win! As minors we could not of course gamble, yet it was perhaps still unwise to teach us *how* to do so!

For the next month I didn't personally come across any major news stories. Though on December the 7th, 2003 I saw throughout all the media (television, radio, newspapers, magazines and billboards) that a 13 year old schoolboy from the Sunshine Coast (Daniel Morcombe) was missing, and there was widespread speculation that he had been abducted. This media story continued for eight whole years with a heartbreaking conclusion. Sadly, what I think affected me most about Daniel's disappearance was that he was due to celebrate his 14th birthday, a mere week after I would celebrate my own. That made the story even more personal and upsetting for me.

Yet I was soon to hear about another major news story that also occurred during December of 2003. This was of Saddam Hussein having been found inside a farmhouse, and within a few years he was trialled and sentenced to be hanged.

That initial news event occurred a few days after my 14th birthday. Elanah had slept over at our house, and we were going to her place later on for a swim, as it was such a hot day. After hearing the news in the morning of Saddam Hussein having been found hidden inside a farmhouse, we did indeed end up going swimming shortly afterward. I put on sunscreen, a shirt and a hat. Though due to the fact of it being such a sunny day and that I had been in the swimming pool for hours, I got severely sunburnt. Due to my mother and her family coming from Northern England, which certainly doesn't experience such intense Queensland sun, my skin is rather fair. As a result of this my sunburn was so bad that my skin was fully blistered and dark purple, which took almost a year to fade entirely.

Thus it was a very sore end to that year, despite having had enjoyable moments in 2003; excluding of course the accidents and injuries which occurred. My hopes for 2004 were that I would have a productive end to middle school. But everything that would come along (both positive and negative) was in no way similar to what I had even imagined to occur.

SECTION THREE

MORE FAMILY AND DIAGNOSES

CHAPTER FIFTEEN

A DEPRESSING TIME WITH POSITIVE DISTRACTIONS

On January the 3rd, 2004 (which was a Saturday) I visited a school friend for the day. We had a fabulous time on their rural property, where there was a lot of yard space. Much of the morning was spent by playing quick songs on the keyboard and talking on some *Harry Potter* forums online. Then after lunch we had a swim in the pool.

It wasn't even a month since my last swim, when I got severely sunburnt, and my skin was still blistered in some places. But I made sure I was well covered with plenty of sunscreen, and I also took care with the amount of time spent in the water.

It ended up being a very enjoyable afternoon, and when my mother picked me up, she even brought along our pet bantam Pigwidgeon (who was named after Ron Weasley's owl in the *Harry Potter* books).

A few weeks later I began Grade Nine at school. At the beginning of that year I was determined that I was going to try my best. Looking back now, I had always tried my best from the very beginning. Though in terms of school my effort was acknowledged solely by my marks.

To begin with I surprised myself, my teachers and mum with very good marks for my schoolwork. This was because I had then imagined it to be a good idea to dedicate my whole time to school, and to not act in any way which was different to what my teachers expected of us students.

Even while I was at home, everything that I verbalised had to strictly be a carbon copy of what I had heard teachers saying at school. Initially I felt that mimicking their actions would enable me to learn exactly what was needed to pass my assessments. Yet this quickly escalated into a manic obsession, which made my mother very concerned.

For instance, there was a time when I had put so much time throughout a week into an assignment, and had gone to bed the night before with a feeling of being so proud that I had finished it. I savoured the thought that I may for the first time have gotten a pass for a major assignment of a semester, which wasn't a weekly homework assessment.

Though I had never hoped for what I actually did get the very next day. The teacher looked at it and gave it the lowest possible grade (in both achievement and effort), wrote a note to my mother saying that I wasn't trying hard enough and I was given a detention for being 'lazy'.

That night after school (once the news of receiving a detention reached home) I had an intense episode. I ended up involuntarily shouting things out to my mum, that I'm certain the whole neighbourhood heard. Poison came spitting out of me which included "When I'm up all night do people think I'm having a party or something"?, "You and my teachers will have gotten more sleep than I did this week, yet I got the same recognition as a lazy person who did absolutely nothing", "I got a detention today for something I personally believe I should have gotten student of the week for, due to all of the hard work I put into that assignment", and "Instead of 'try harder Rebecca' why can't any person say well done for the effort, Rebecca"?.

My mother was initially shocked that I was speaking (or more rather yelling) to her in this manner, and afterwards I felt so ashamed and embarrassed about the words that were rushing out of my mouth. But afterward she hugged me and gently said "I'm so sorry sweetie, I know exactly how you feel".

At school I wasn't coping well with anything else either. I had completely lost interest in socialising with anyone and had become obsessed with my school work. This obsession was to the point where I never thought of anything else but school, I was constantly dreaming about my homework, and had realised that I was always reciting my lessons out loud while I was sleeping. Thus it didn't take long for my obsession to turn into depression.

In a metaphorical sense depression is very much like a blackhole. Each and every person has a susceptibility to depression by their own personal triggers. We begin to feel the effects of the metaphorical blackhole as excessive stress. A similarity is that both blackholes and the formation of depression have an event horizon where once we enter there's no way of naturally escaping it's pull.

I've now discovered that my primary trigger for depression is when I feel that I'm being accused of not trying hard enough. That has been the case all the way through my life so far. In the early months of 2004 I was conscious of putting 100% effort into my schoolwork, because I didn't want another year of getting into trouble for not passing an assignment.

Yet I felt that I wasn't succeeding, and being constantly told to try harder made me feel more pressured, and as if I wasn't being acknowledged for the intense effort that I was putting in. In simpler terms, it essentially made me feel like I was getting accused of being lazy.

As I spiralled deeper into depression I was back to having trouble sleeping at night. I did fear the sun rising before I fell asleep, just as I had done five years previously. However, by this time I had many additional fears, which included a fear of dying whenever I fell asleep.

Despite knowing that it was completely irrational, I feared that I may lose my ability to wake up, and I felt that the more fatigued I was when I fell asleep meant that there was a stronger likelihood of this happening. So my combined anxiety/fatigue from the sleeping issues and the pressure from school meant that I wasn't in a healthy state of mind at all.

I must too add that it is so much easier for me, whenever I have a sleepless night in the current day. Back in 2004 there were no streaming sites where I could watch whatever I wanted on my television.

It's true that most free to air channels broadcasted shows and movies 24/7. However late night television never had shows that I wanted to watch, and nor were most of them appropriate for children and adolescents to watch. Firstly, there were many sexual commercials and con artists trying to sell useless products. Many presenters in those late night informercials spoke by using extremely weird voices and expressions that I found very creepy.

Also, there were emotionally brainwashing televangelist shows, as well as shows about demonic exorcisms. For example, there was a time when I made a mistake of turning the television on in the middle of the night.

Unfortunately a show was being aired which featured a young girl who was supposedly possessed by the devil. She had foam coming out of her mouth and was screaming and jeering, while holy water and a cross were being thrown on top of her. The priest was also yelling at this girl and violently shaking her, which frightened me very much.

So as a result of all that, the option of watching television on a sleepless night definitely wasn't possible in those days. There was the occasional DVD to watch but options were very limited, and once a movie was watched over and over again it would no longer relax me.

In regards to the internet, there was Myspace and Facebook. Though social media was no where near as good or easy to access as it is today. Minecraft didn't yet exist (which I now use as a relaxing game), there were no eBooks and the games which were then available didn't at all relax me. Additionally, in order to play one of those games I would have to turn the whole computer system on, and therefore wake up everyone in the house.

Thus, whenever I was still awake in the early hours of the morning, it truly did feel as if I was the only person alive in a world that was abandoned. Everything was eerily quiet, sinister and my imagination would make the night seem even darker. I definitely didn't enjoy sleepless nights back in those days.

From the age of three I had been receiving psychotherapy for my depression and anxiety. Though it was being treated as a temporary aid that I would only need for a few years. So my doctor said throughout my childhood that he didn't want me on medication for my anxiety. This was because he wanted me to learn how to handle the anxiety attacks on my own (without medication) before I presumably outgrew them.

Yet by that stage it came to a point where mum felt that she needed to express to him more strongly that there was something else going on here. She said that I wasn't sleeping well at all. Every night I had next to no sleep, was afraid to be in my own bed (depression often makes a person regress back to younger years), or was yelling and crying out loud in my sleep. Mum was in a position where she felt guilty about sending me to school each day while I was in that state of mind. So she said to my doctor that I needed to be on medication, as psychotherapy alone would not be able to solve this.

I was first put on Temazepam to help me sleep at night. However the way it would make me rapidly fall into a deep sleep increased my fears of not being able to wake up again. Then I was put on Zoloft instead to aid my depression. For a very brief time it worked successfully. The depression and irrational fears left me, even though I was still struggling with my schoolwork. My doctor (who I'm keeping anonymous) was happy about this, and he agreed with both Mum and I that daily medication would perhaps be needed permanently. He also diagnosed me with Performance Anxiety Disorder (which we now know wasn't a fully accurate diagnosis) and gave my teachers a medical note saying that I shouldn't be pressured to work harder.

However, if I take away my problems with sleeping and issues related to my schoolwork, 2004 certainly wasn't a disastrous year overall. There were indeed some very enjoyable life experiences, including the expansion of our tiny family of three.

In May of 2004 mum met my stepdad, Brent and his three children Kylie, Brendan and Dylan. Jessica and I first met Brent, Kylie (then aged 7) and Brendan (then aged 5) at Warner Brothers Movie World on Saturday June the 19th of that year (6 days after Kylie's 7th birthday). Though Mum and Brent had first met each other at the Greenbank RSL a few months prior to then.

We had an enjoyable day, which was spent mainly at Loony Toons Village. Afterward Brent took Kylie and Brendan back to their mother's house, and Mum took me and Jessica to a dine-in takeaway restaurant. There we spoke about how we liked Brent and his two oldest children very much. We met (then) two year old Dylan a month later on Saturday July the 10th. Dylan was a really pleasant child as well.

For much of that year we spent our weekends getting to know each other, by going down to Brent's house where we were a family of seven.

This was prior to Brent and his three children coming to live with us in our present day home. We always had a very enjoyable time each and every weekend, and once the weather became warmer it was nice to have a swim in the pool.

It was a fortunate coincidence that Brent's three children were then being assessed for various kinds of disabilities. One of the main reasons for why this was so fortunate is that mum at the time was seriously considering to get me assessed for certain conditions, including autism and Obsessive Compulsive Disorder.

In regards to her concerns about me having Obsessive Compulsive Disorder, there was an episode I had later in 2004, which was perhaps triggered by my stress from school. On Halloween we were going down to the Gold Coast for a family get together (Mum, me and Jessica with Brent, Kylie, Brendan and Dylan). Mum bought some sausages for the younger kids. Yet definitely not for me because I detest the taste of sausage meat.

Anyhow they ended up remaining uneaten in the fridge for nearly three weeks, and when my mother had them on the kitchen bench to give to the dog I was petrified of them. I had no idea they were still in the house and I didn't sleep that night as a result. It was so frightening how the preservatives made them look so normal, with all the poison and bacteria masked. The memory of seeing those sausages gave me years of nightmares, and the memory of them today still gives me goosebumps.

It would be a few more years until I got diagnosed with Obsessive Compulsive Disorder (that created my fear of dangerous food) and Highly Superior Autobiographical Memory (which caused this memory to permanently stay with me). Yet despite not yet having a diagnosis of those two conditions, they still affected my life to the exact same level regardless.

The next year, 2005 was essentially a continuation of what began for me the previous year. My relationship with my new step-family became much closer (and the word 'step' could then be removed from 'family'), and my family's persistence towards me getting an autism diagnosis finally reached a successful conclusion.

CHAPTER SIXTEEN

IT'S NOW KNOWN THAT I HAVE AUTISM

In December of 2004 I celebrated my 15th birthday at Dreamworld with my family and a couple of school friends. On the previous day (Friday December the 10th, 2004) it was pouring down with rain in Southeast Queensland and the bad weather was expected to continue through to the next day. That worried us because there was a possibility that my birthday celebration at Dreamworld may have had to be cancelled.

Yet a family friend had given me a 'protective charm' bracelet as an early birthday present on Friday evening, prior to having dinner together at Sizzler. The bracelet was made of carnelian and tigers eye and I liked the sensation of the stones on my skin. I've always liked the way that crystals and rocks feel when I run my hands over the texture of them. It's also very nice to own a box of them to tangibly sort through for many hours.

Later that night I was very tired, so I was in a hurry to get to bed. I ended up sleeping in the clothes I was wearing, which included the bracelet. For all I know, the bracelet could have been full of luck, because when I awoke the following morning the sun was shining and all of the previous day's cloud had disappeared; or else it was likely due to weather reports decades ago not being quite so accurate. But regardless my friends immediately rang me up at breakfast time, as they were so excited about the fact that we could go to Dreamworld after all!

That day we had a great deal of fun. The character Spongebob sang Happy Birthday to me in Nickelodeon Central, we had pizza for lunch, ice-cream as an afternoon snack, and then came home to have some birthday cake.

Two weeks later we had a great Christmas together as a family. Brent was determined to make it the best Christmas that the five of us kids had ever had. We had a heap of presents to open at mum's house (where we currently live), and then we opened our second half down at Brent's house. After a fabulous afternoon with all of his family (me, mum and Jessica weren't in contact with any of our blood relatives at that time) I finally went to bed at 11pm happy, very tired and full of delicious food.

We returned to mum's house the following morning, and unfortunately heard breaking news of a massive earthquake that had happened in the Indian Ocean in the early hours of the morning. That earthquake generated tsunamis and devastation in multiple countries. South East Asia is a very popular place for Australian tourists as it's so close to home. There are also many people from those affected countries who emigrate to Australia, or visit as tourists themselves. So there was rolling coverage of this disaster across all of our media, and everybody within Australia was strongly advised to not travel to South East Asian seaside destinations at that time. This was just in case there were aftershocks from the earthquake and/or further tsunamis.

Though, at the very end of December, Brent brought home a surprise which was pleasant news for us all. As an early birthday present for Mum he got her a new puppy named Samson. Sparky had long since been the only dog living in the house, and she didn't take a liking to Sam immediately. She was fine with cats, but every time Sam would approach her she would growl at him.

Samson was a small but tough little ShihTzu, despite technically being half chihuahua. At that time we didn't believe that he had any chihuahua in him at all. In February of the following year we got a female Maltese named Buffy to keep him company. Therefore I had a relaxing lead up to my return to school, as I had puppies to train and play games with.

The next school year (Grade Ten) was when I moved up into the senior sub school at Calamvale. Previously I had been in the middle school and was initially excited about moving into the area which had the best facilities. Calamvale Community College was in the process of being built as I was moving up through the grades. So the senior school was the newest area and had a cafe, walk-in canteen and a performing arts theatre with a nice foyer. It was a novelty to be there at first, but unfortunately it wasn't long before I took that all for granted.

As it was a new school year for me, the medical letter written by my doctor was no longer valid. So I was back to having full expectations in regards to my school work. Initially I thought I was managing myself well, as I was getting B grades and higher. This satisfied me because I was no longer getting the lowest marks in the class. So I felt like I was finally making progress.

However it didn't take long for the work I was being set to change. Each class was giving us unexpected assignments with very short deadlines. Thus I'd be set three 500 word+ essays each and every week, in addition to other kinds of assessments. It is true that I have always enjoyed writing. But the teachers no longer wanted me to write out factual information. They again wanted me to study and discuss the reasons for everything that wasn't black and white. I would still complete all of my homework to the best of my ability. Yet I'd get a D grade every time because it didn't fit the exact criteria that the teachers were asking for.

Assignments were coming along constantly, and I was doing my best to keep up with them all, but due dates came and went before I had even finished them. The fact that I was working so hard yet getting the lowest marks possible was giving me so much stress and anxiety.

I was given no extra assistance at all, and whenever I asked my teachers for help, I was unable to understand what they were telling me. At that time mum was still unaware of my (exact) learning difficulties, despite doing everything that she could to help me.

By then she was questioning whether the negative results from my first autism assessment were indeed true. But the doctor I was seeing regularly told us that he did not believe I was autistic in any way, and that this extra depression I was experiencing was merely due to teenage hormones.

Both Mum and myself emphatically said that the stress was due to the pressure of being set an astronomical amount of work that I simply could not do, regardless of the time and effort I was putting in to complete each task. Though my doctor said that he would increase my dosage of Zoloft and assured us that once the anxiety was gone I would be able to complete my school work with ease.

Though increasing the Zoloft only made things worse. Zoloft was keeping me up until the early hours of the morning, and whenever I fell asleep and woke up I would experience severe episodes of Sleep Paralysis. With that I would be immobile with my eyelids shut and/or continuing a dream up to a whole minute after opening my eyes.

I would experience this on a nightly basis, and would try to ease myself through it by reminding myself that it was harmless. However it's always very difficult to do so while I am in the middle of an experience which is so uncomfortable and frightening. In fact as a young child I would hold my eyelids open in the middle of the night, or I would deliberately move around in bed with the hope that I could prevent myself from falling asleep, as I would most probably experience Sleep Paralysis again.

After an episode of Sleep Paralysis I either start dreaming again, or I may eventually force my eyes open; which are sometimes even still darting around for a minute or two, as they do in REM (or Rapid Eye Movement) Sleep. As a result of this happening constantly with the increase of the Zoloft, I was getting barely any sleep each and every night during that time.

So in summary the extra medication that I was given didn't take away my depression and anxiety, and it certainly didn't enable me to get pass marks for my school work. After reading all of what was said above, one could assume that the year 2005 was disastrous for me overall. But that wasn't at all true.

It was evident that it was school which was causing all of my problems, because on weekends and school holidays I was experiencing no characteristics of depression whatsoever. In fact I had many occasions at home during that year when I thoroughly enjoyed myself. For our first Easter together (as a family of seven) we were given an Xbox with a couple of games. Predictably, there wasn't a moment when at least a few of us didn't want to use the Xbox. So we'd be given a set amount of time (on any non-school day) to play on it.

During the middle of 2005 we also went to a few of the Big Brother

Eviction Shows. The Australian version of *Big Brother* was originally filmed at a studio-house located within Dreamworld. The live shows were filmed in front of an audience at Dreamworld Studios. On Sunday May the 22nd me, mum and Brent saw the first eviction show of that year. This wasn't initially planned either. We as a family went to Dreamworld that day and they were selling last minute tickets for the show that night.

Big Brother was something we enjoyed watching on television, but we had never been to a live show before. So we bought a few tickets, just so we could see what it was like before taking the younger kids along. We ended up liking the experience enormously, and on Sunday June the 5th we took Kylie, Brendan and Dylan along with us to another eviction show.

This was an early birthday present for Kylie (who was to turn eight on June the 13th). Eviction shows were something we greatly enjoyed, yet didn't have enough money to go to every week.

But luckily the Greenbank RSL Club, which is walking distance from our house, held *Big Brother* Eviction parties on Sunday nights. They had the show playing live in (what was then) the lounge area. In addition to that, the evictee from the previous week was there in person. These shows were free to attend as well.

There was another hobby that I had commenced that year, which I ended up staying with far longer than I did with dancing. In fact I do still practice it to this very day.

The year 2005 was when I began doing Taekwondo. This was decided on by my parents, as they felt that it would help to build my self-confidence, and be a good way to reduce my stress levels from school. Brent by that time was a Red Belt Three Stripe (one rank before provisional black belt). I ended up liking Taekwondo a lot, and by the year's end I had done three gradings, getting to Yellow Belt Three Stripe.

Brent, Kylie and Brendan attended classes with me, and that was a great way to quickly bond as a family. Yet my family and step-family began merging together as one in other ways too.

During this year one of Brent's sons (then four year old Dylan) came to live with us full time because his biological mother felt that he was an absolute handful to raise and look after. Though I can now say, after personally living with Dylan for over fifteen years, that the truth is that he has never had behaviour problems of any kind.

So the large patio in the back garden had to be converted into a bedroom and living room for our parents, while Dylan was to move into their previous bedroom. Despite the fact that he was then aged four, Dylan had never before had a bedroom.

Initially he was a baby sleeping in a crib within his siblings' room. Then after his parents' divorce his biological mother had managed to put him into foster care, without Brent's knowledge. Thus he had been moved around from house to house for a couple of years. Of course, it didn't take long for Brent to discover that Dylan had been sent away. However it was a struggle for Brent to remove Dylan from foster care (as Dylan himself talks about as a young man in our 2022 film). But when he eventually came to live with us he finally had his very own bedroom. To mark that occasion mum painted his bedroom (just like she had done with my *Harry Potter* room) in the theme of a popular Australian children's show of the time, *The Wiggles*.

Dylan loved and appreciated this so much. His verbal skills were very limited, yet he expressed all of his messages of thanks by kissing each individual wall.

At that time Dylan was getting assessed for autism and Intellectual Impairment, which he ended up being diagnosed with. Yet while mum was reading leaflets and articles about autism, which were sent to her from Autism Queensland, the first person who came to mind as she was going through all of the descriptive material was myself. So she lent me all of the leaflets and articles to read.

As I was reading through them all, I was given so much insight into various things which I had always lived with. I had known for a long time that I had characteristics which were different from most people. Everyone else I had met at home and at school knew so too, and that was why I had always experienced bullying from time to time.

Yet, up until then I hadn't known that it was autism. Instead I had felt that I was some kind of 'freak', that nobody else but me had those issues, and that 'Rebecca Sharrock' was the most undesirable and lamest person in the world. At that time I felt so low that I hated to hear my very name, as well as to think about every other part of how I existed.

However after reading through this material I came to an inner conclusion that I must have had autism, and I had a positive belief that a diagnosis would end that chapter of confusion for me. My parents felt so too and my mother expressed this to my doctor. He did agree that the way my challenges and anxiety were not being helped after increasing the Zoloft was unusual, as was my inability to properly use a knife and fork (which my mother had expressed to him). Hand-eye coordination and dexterity skills continue to be a struggle to this day.

However he unexpectedly told us that he wanted me tested for bipolar disorder. When it came to his suggestion of me having bipolar disorder, mum expressed to him that I was only ever experiencing the same kind of anxiety, and was never having swings between different kinds of emotions.

Mum said that she firmly believed that I had autism and that she wanted me re-assessed for it. He finally said that it would be a good idea to get me assessed, in order for us to rule out the possibility that I had autism.

When I went to have my second assessment for autism (after my first at the age of six) the results were very clean-cut. On my very first meeting with the psychologist we were told that she was 100% certain that I had autism. She also said that it was so unfortunate that this finally got recognised so late in my school years. Me and mum both fully agreed. Though we were informed that this was quite a common occurrence for autistic females of my time.

Yet by saying all of that, we were also told that I had an enormous amount of the traditional, significant and obvious characteristics of autism. This made it incredible for her to hear that I had missed an earlier diagnosis, regardless of my gender.

Autistic females may not be (or appear to be) quite as socially awkward as autistic males. My own guess (merely based upon my own individual experience) is that there are many more expectations placed upon females in the areas that autism affects. These include having extra social skills, quicker processing abilities, and (in particular) an exemplary understanding of complex emotions. Many autistic people have enormous difficulty in coping with and even understanding those kinds of things.

In order to fit in many autistic females can at first mask and bluff their way through social and emotional challenges. But we can only make that work effectively for a certain amount of time. Once we reach our teen years this no longer works. This is due to the fact that by that time, most females have developed more social and emotional abilities than many autistic people generally have the capacity for. As a result a fair number of people (including myself) struggle greatly with experiencing that enormous level of pressure; and this causes a lot of anxiety, stress and depressive feelings. Personally, I feel that this is more likely the cause for autistic females often having attached anxiety disorders, rather than it coming from hormone fluctuations. This is also evident when we see many autistic people who aren't female having an equivalent amount of anxiety.

It was also during that assessment when the suggestion of doing writing as a career was first given to me. My psychologist was telling us that many autistic people had a passion for writing. This was said after I answered her question about what I liked to do in my spare time.

Despite her making this observation of me, I had never before thought about making a career for myself as a writer, nor had I thought of myself as having enough skill in any area whatsoever for a career. But I had the story of Donna Williams (a popular autistic writer, speaker and advocate of the time and still to this day) explained to me. This gave me a huge amount of inspiration and encouragement.

So now we had achieved the goal of successfully getting a diagnosis of autism from an assessment. However the following year was when I had to adjust my whole life to accommodate what I had just been diagnosed with. I was soon to find out that it would be nowhere near as smooth a task as I had initially expected.

CHAPTER SEVENTEEN

WHERE DO I GO TO FROM HERE?

Just over a month later, on December the 11th, 2005 I had my 16th birthday. First thing in the morning I woke up to hear some additional news. Our dog Buffy, who was pregnant with her first litter of puppies, had gone into labor. While I was receiving all of my cards and gifts, we were also giving the dog attention and making her feel comfortable. Me and the rest of the family thought that it was superb to share my birthday with those puppies!

Buffy was due to be in labor for a good few hours, so it was safe to leave her alone for a short while; just as long as she was comfortable in our parents' living room and that the other two dogs were locked outside with some food and water. My parents were adamant that all of the plans for this milestone birthday would not be canceled.

We spent most of that morning out at the shops and we had Sizzler for lunch. Then in the late afternoon we came home to have my birthday cake, which mum had made to look like the Hogwarts Express from *Harry Potter*.

Afterward we spent our evening with Buffy who was finally giving birth to her puppies. Buffy had only just turned one year old on the previous day. Thus she was very young in addition to being a small Maltese. She took a long time to give birth and was in incredible pain, so we called a vet expressing our concerns. We were then told to wait another hour and a half, and if she hadn't had any of her puppies by then we were to take her to our local veterinary hospital.

Luckily by the time we put the phone down her three puppies came out one by one.

I must add here that this was her only litter of which she showed any nurturing connection towards. Buffy would growl at Samson whenever he wanted to come in for a peek. Though our oldest dog Sparky showed such surprising intelligence and agility on that first night. Sparky was supposed to be completely blind with severe arthritis, and would slowly hobble around the house. Yet in the middle of the night she sneaked out of her bed, jumped up onto the back of the long sofa barricading the puppies, quickly scaled along the edge in pitch black darkness, and went in for a nosy as to what was going on. Little did she know that Brent had seen the whole thing and said "If I hadn't actually seen that I would never have believed it"!

For Christmas two weeks later I got a heap of craft and hobby equipment to start building what was originally going to be a *Harry Potter* railway set (I later turned it into a *Harry Potter* Lego Village). As for the rest of our family's presents Jessica got a first generation Nintendo DS, Kylie got a dollhouse and the boys got a radio control car each.

On a much bleaker note however, I'd have to say that the year 2006 was the most difficult twelve months of my life. On every day of 2006 I felt thoroughly miserable and didn't see the point of living my life at all. I still had a few happy experiences, yet at those times an undertone of the depression mentioned above still lingered.

We were assured by the school at the end of the previous year that I would have a teacher aide supporting me in every class. On my first day back at school however, we discovered that they hadn't told us the truth. I had no assistance in any class, didn't have an IEP (Individual Education Plan) either explained or arranged, and my teachers hadn't even been informed that I had just been diagnosed with learning difficulties.

Mum was absolutely disgusted, and we went up to the admin after school in the hope of getting an explanation as to why this had happened. The answer we were given was that they had previously misinformed us. We were told that I wasn't allowed to have an IEP in my senior years due to the fact that they believed it would be unfair for the neurotypical students without challenges.

Yet the reality was that they made it unfair for students *with* challenges. It's true for those of us with disabilities that other areas often compensate, by giving us abilities in different places. Though the school curriculum and society (especially at that time) mostly required cognitive skills which I lacked, and all of the areas where I had strengths were of little to no use in school and/or the world in general.

Also, we were told that the last thing they'd want would be for the majority of their students to fail school. But they couldn't care less about the minority of students with challenges (including myself) failing school as a result of that decision.

In recent years a few ignorant members of the public have brought up a theory that neurotypical students are being brought down in their grades, as a result of the standard of work being lowered to cater for special needs students. That theory is absolute rubbish. Those of us who have disabilities are (and always have been, to this current day) marginalised in all areas of general society. As well, the reason for why I struggled in class was because the work *wasn't* catered towards students like myself with learning difficulties.

Contrary to what a few have said to me as well, having students with learning difficulties flounder in a mainstream classroom (back in the year 2006, anyhow) without any kind of support is not at all inclusion. It wasn't in any way enjoyable or fulfilling to be spending each and every lesson staring at a white wall, and to not understand any of the work I was supposed to be doing. Communication was difficult for me, but even when I was able to ask questions for clarification, I was still unable to comprehend any of the words which I had received.

Of course this doesn't necessarily mean that we're completely excluded. Yet society is primarily designed and structured for the needs and desires of people who are neurotypical (especially a decade and a half ago). It's understandable that it's much easier to cater for the interests of the majority of our population. Yet the rest us with disabilities are still living beings who didn't choose to be in this situation.

Despite having been known to have anxiety all throughout my school career (and I wasn't ever given an IEP for my anxiety) it was assumed that my late autism diagnosis meant that I needed very little assistance. So my case was considered to be of low priority to the school. They also said to us that I wasn't eligible to use their Special Education Unit as I didn't live in a suburb that was termed a catchment area, even though we lived a mere seven minute drive from the school.

In senior school the lessons were an hour and a half long. For most of my classes I would sit through that time stressed, bored and anxious because I was unable to complete any of the work. The work was even harder than the previous year, and most of my teachers didn't have much experience teaching sixteen year olds cognitive skills that are usually gained before primary school age.

The school was also informed that I needed to have ten minute breaks every half hour during class, as the lessons were unusually long (being ninety minutes each). I was supposed to be supervised while having those breaks. Yet most of my teachers responded by sending me outside to wander around the school grounds until I was ready to come back into the classroom.

Though at the same time it wouldn't be fair to not include my favourite Year 11 teachers. My favourite subject by far was maths. This is somewhat surprising as the middle school assignments that kept me up all night were those where I had to talk about numbers and statistics on spreadsheets for that very subject. However senior maths was much more enjoyable for me. We got to primarily do algebra, geometry, trigonometry, and (my personal favourite) global positioning. In fact when I sat an exam on global positioning in term three of that year, I received my first ever A+ grade. My teacher was so happy about that and he made sure I knew during recess before the lesson started.

Also, throughout that year I had a hobby of collecting antique and vintage books. These I would read whenever I felt distressed at school. I always find that stories (in both children's and adults' books) from the victorian era have such a warm and comforting feel. When I brought them to school, I always read them during recess. Many students and teachers (especially my English and Modern History teacher) were in absolute awe of them.

My English teacher was always so happy to see me and other teenagers who enjoyed reading. She also fully understood that I had autism and anxiety. Unfortunately she was forced by Education Queensland to teach her class by the set curriculum. However she knew how hard it was for me to sit in the classroom for ninety minutes whilst being unable to do any of the work. So she lent me one of her antique books to read during class. It was a 19th century medical dictionary, which I was very interested in reading because diseases such as smallpox (which is understood to be fully extinct now) were described in such quaint victorian jargon.

During that year there was a lot going on outside of school too. A mere few months after I was diagnosed with autism, I saw Jason McElwain's story on television. Jason was an autistic high school student and he had a passion for basketball. His incredible talent had been overlooked and he had been placed in his school's reserve team. Yet when he was finally able to play in the game, he achieved score after score which resulted in a clear win for his school. His story was a huge inspiration to me, as it was proof that having autism doesn't make achieving our dreams and following our passions impossible.

In February I was transferred to a psychiatrist who was a lot more experienced (in the field of autism). So I began seeing him for all of my therapy sessions. My medication got readjusted. I stopped taking Zoloft and took Anafranil instead. Anafranil is much better for me, because in addition to being an antidepressant it also takes experiences of sleep paralysis away. We were told that Anafranil had been around since the 1960s and was occasionally used by veterinarians to calm distressed animals. I was also prescribed Lexapro alongside it, just to counteract the unneeded side-effects.

At the beginning of September 2006 I was diagnosed with Obsessive Compulsive Disorder (OCD). That eventual diagnosis mainly came about because throughout that year I had developed a fear about burglars breaking in at night, and murdering me as I slept. For that reason I would pile every single brick we had against the front gate each night, and then I would barricade my bedroom door with a heap of chairs. Mum expressed this to my psychiatrist, along with a few other things (some of them previously mentioned in earlier chapters of this book) and he diagnosed me with OCD.

In regards to my OCD, both mum and I were told that there were many times in my life when bad luck didn't help me very much. It's not that I'm always unlucky and unfortunate. But there have been many moments in my lifetime when things that seemingly confirm my worst fears have unexpectedly and uninvitingly come along to me. My psychiatrist at that time noticed this even quicker than I myself did.

For example, there was a day when he asked me about whether there ever had been a time when a source other than my own thoughts had given me proof that my fears were realistic.

I answered by telling him that there had been an occasion when I walked through the living room one evening in 2004, and caught a news story about a girl who woke up to find that both of her parents had unexpectedly died in their sleep. Unluckily that was also during the time when I had fears of losing the ability to wake up.

My psychiatrist then said that the media often dramatise stories in the hope of engaging their viewers' interest. Yet I told him that it was definitely true, and he asked me how I knew that. Then I explained to him that we received a phone call the next day from one of me and my sister's close school friends, and discovered that *she* was the girl whose parents had died in that news story. We knew her family so well that we would regularly visit them at their house.

Though at the time of her call about her parents' death, she was in the care of extended family and she was inviting us to her parents' funeral. We attended the service on October the 4th of that year, and discovered through an autopsy that the father had died in his sleep due to underlying health conditions, then the mother had a fatal heart attack after finding him dead.

I also told my psychiatrist that there were several other moments in 2005 and 2006 when I would turn my television on, and there would unexpectedly be a news story about an out of control car crashing into a person's bedroom or house overnight, and occasionally bursting into flames (that was my nightly fear during those two years). These were the days when televisions would initially be set to the most recent channel that the aerial was tuned into, and we would have to change channels with a remote once the television was turned on again.

My psychiatrist did fully believe me and knew that these weren't dramatised stories coming from hysteria. However he did express to my mother and I that due to a combination of OCD and bad luck, it was essential for me not to turn my television on during times when the daily news was showing.

He also arranged for me to be put on Xyprexa. That was very hard to get a prescription for in 2006. Yet my previous psychiatrist (who we were still in contact with at that early time) arranged with success for me to get prescribed with Xyprexa as soon as possible. My previous psychiatrist was very apologetic about his mistake and neither me nor my family hold any hard feelings against him. Anyone can make mistakes, my issues of past trauma made it more challenging for me to get a diagnosis of autism, and of course not as much was known about autism a decade or two ago.

Though it was very good to finally receive (most of) the answers to my mental health and cognitive difficulties, from a diagnosis of both autism and Obsessive Compulsive Disorder. As well, the combination/blending of my family and step-family also became fully fixed at roughly the same time. The year 2006 was when Brendan (then aged 7) and Kylie (then aged 9) came to live with us full time. Their biological mother who had been diagnosed with Intellectual Impairment and autism found parenting too hard a job. To this day she has not been in contact with us, and many strangers who have been seeing her more recently have been very surprised to hear from us that she had ever become a parent. The latest we've heard about her whereabouts is that she is now living in a local SIL (Supported Independent Living) house with a carer. Though at least Kylie, Brendan and Dylan got to live a good childhood whilst being raised by Mum and Brent.

Dylan turned five on September the 18th and he got a large tank full of pet fish for his birthday. He spent a lot of time looking at them, and there was a time when he pointed one of the fish out to us, that had a white stripe on its tail. It was merely swimming through one of the ornaments in the tank, just like any innocent pet fish would. But Dylan (despite his severe verbal language delay) literally said "See that fish there. Get rid of that fish. I don't like him, because he's a bully". When the fish passed away a year and a half later, his Grandma (who taught Sunday School to children at her local church) told him that it had gone to heaven. Dylan then said "Not heaven. Only good people go to heaven". His grandma of course was shocked to hear those words.

Unlike Jessica and I, Brent's three children got to see a lot of their grandparents whilst growing up. Many a time this would make me feel a little envious inside.

However, during the following month of that year (October 2006) something rather strange and unexpected happened. I was playing Crash Bandicoot on my Xbox, and mum knocked on my door and asked me "Do you want to say hello to Grandad"?

This was extremely bizarre as we had heard nothing at all from him since I was eight. In fact it felt very much like meeting someone alive, after attending their funeral many years before. When I entered the living room he stared at me for a minute without saying anything. He looked almost exactly the same as he did when I had last seen him eight years prior to then, and the only difference was that he'd gathered a few more white hairs. Then I broke the silence by saying "Hi, Grandad". Verbalising the word 'grandad' was strange to me because it had been eight years since I had said that. Grandad responded by simply saying "You're beautiful".

Grandad also mentioned how he had divorced our nana a little while ago and had met a woman (Diane) online. They had been friends in England when they were seventeen, but had lost contact when they'd gone their own ways in life. Diane had emigrated to Canada and Grandad had brought nana, mum and my aunt along to Australia in 1973. Though as they had again met, Grandad told us he was getting married to Diane and would be moving over to Canada to live with her.

October 2006 was also a significant part of my life because it was the time when I had finally understood what I was told exactly a year earlier, which was about me doing writing as a career. Each and every day I would constantly go over my life experiences. So one night when I came home from Taekwondo class, I got into the shower and came to the realisation that I *should* write a book about all of the things I constantly pondered over. Thus I initially began by writing a small book called Living With Aspergers Syndrome. Aspergers Syndrome was formerly a branch of autism. But branches of autism such as Aspergers and PDD-NOS have now all been classified as Autism Spectrum Disorder. Now the terms High Functioning Autism and Low Functioning Autism have also been phased out. We've been told during seminars that it's best to say "autism with high support needs" and "autism with low support needs". Yet each individual person has their own preference, and terminology changes all the time. Everything said previously in this paragraph is correct to 2021.

So the year 2006 began in a very awkward way for me. Yet this was to be expected as it was the time when me, my family and my school were adjusting to the knowledge that I had autism. But as I moved towards 2007 the situation had really started to settle, and then my life wasn't quite as difficult as it was the previous year.

CHAPTER EIGHTEEN

TRAVELING FORWARD INTO NEW BEGINNINGS

A short while later, in December of 2006, I enjoyed my birthday as usual. My presents included an electronic keyboard, a sports watch and a box of *Harry Potter* stickers. That day Jessica made me some pancakes for breakfast, Dylan graduated from kindergarten, and we went out to buy some antique records for mum's 'new' gramophone. Afterward we had dinner and cake at home.

Two weeks later we enjoyed our first Christmas together as a family of seven people (who were living under one roof). We each got a radio control car as a present and we spent much of the day at our local park racing them. Brent's radio control car was of course the best one, as it could top 110km/h (68mph) and was powered by petrol. The rest of us had rechargeable cars yet it was much easier to find extra additions for those, such as drift tyres.

Mum had her gramophone playing for most of the day too. She had purchased an antique record which played the song 'The Man On The Flying Trapeze' from an antique shop. Unfortunately though, Grandad did put a large scratch on it when he incorrectly stopped the turntable before lifting up the needle. Therefore one side of the record (and the first part of the entire song) is sadly unplayable now. Yet at least the second half of the song still plays beautifully.

The next year (2007) was a little easier than the previous one, even though I wasn't completely out of the woods because I was still at school. A few days into January we were having dinner at a family friend's house and I was asked about what I hoped the new year would bring along. My answer was plainly and simply "I hope it will be better than last year". Everyone at the table jokingly said that my response was a very cliché goal for a new year. Yet regardless of whether that was the case or not, my response was the absolute truth.

In December of 2006 my mother had told the school that if they didn't cater for my needs during my final year, she would have no other option but to pull me out. So we were reassured that it wouldn't be like the previous year, I would have learning support in each class, my work would be adjusted to my needs, and that they would use my English lessons as time to work on my book.

We were told as well that I didn't have to be at school for the first day back. However we received a phone call by the school that afternoon, which was them querying us as to why I was absent on that day. Mum then asked "Didn't you say that she wasn't required to be at school today"? She was then told that everything they said previously was just to stop her from pulling me out of school.

So Mum asked about whether I'd have support in the classroom and whether my assessments would be specifically structured as promised; and their answer was that they couldn't do that.

Then Mum actually told them there and then that if they fell back on their promise and gave me a year like the previous one, she would take further action. That's when they gave a genuine promise of catering my final school year to my needs.

In my adjusted IEP I only had to attend maths class and art class without additional support, as those were the subjects that I didn't mind too much. Though I did history and English in a quiet room with a support teacher. With history and English, the work I was doing was adjusted to my capabilities. This did of course mean that I couldn't get any qualifications from school itself. However it did give me a good head start on my process of catching up on the skills I missed during my time at school. That process continued well into my twenties.

At the beginning of the year I watched the film *Bowling For Columbine* in English class. As the story of students being killed by two of their fellow pupils was so horrific, I previously believed that it was merely a fictional movie. Back in the year 1999 (when the Columbine massacre occurred) my mother didn't allow me to watch the news, as she correctly believed that I was too young to cope with stories like this.

Though on Monday April the 16th, I coincidently woke up to the news of the Virginia Tech massacre. It was then when I was struck with the realisation that the Columbine massacre was indeed real (as was mentioned in this 2007 news report), and that there *were* horrific shootings like this happening within our world! The news of that shocked and saddened me greatly.

For the second semester of my final school year, I watched and did a written assessment for the movie *The Green Mile* (this time for history). It was a movie that my mother had liked when it came out. Yet the only part that mum had allowed me to watch as a child was when John Coffey gave the prison warder Paul Edgecomb his healing power. During that school term I watched the whole film, and in truth I quite enjoyed it. Yet it's not the type of movie I'd personally enjoy watching again and again, purely because there are some very intense topics involved.

On the other hand though, the *Harry Potter* movies are the sort that I can enjoy watching again and again. The film *Harry Potter and the Order of the Phoenix* was released in Australian cinemas on July the 25th of that year. As was our tradition with all of the *Harry Potter* films, we went to see the first screening of it at our local cinema.

The very next day (which was a Thursday) my friend Monica dropped by at our house to see me. We talked for a few hours and then came up with the idea of seeing the new *Harry Potter* movie together. Monica's two youngest sisters came along as well. By the time we arrived at the cinema however, we found out that the movie had started twenty minutes beforehand. So prior to watching the next screening, we ended up having McDonalds for dinner at the mall.

Once we were eventually in the cinema, we all enjoyed watching the film. During the scene where Bellatrix Lestrange was struggling out of chains in her Azkaban mugshot (Azkaban is a fictional prison in the *Harry Potter* series), we burst out laughing at her twisted face whilst she was yelling. In the world of *Harry Potter*, photos don't stay still in their frames. They're more rather like small television or computer screens, which are powered by magic and not electricity of course.

A few days later however, I didn't have nearly as great of a day. I woke up to the news that Sparky was terminally ill and had incurable pain. So we had no choice but to take her to the vet to get euthanised. Losing Sparky happened so unexpectedly that it was nearly a month before the horrible truth settled in for me. She had after all been my beloved pet dog since I was five years old. Yet I gradually adjusted to life without Sparky, and I still have her collar and tag stored in a special place to this day. But despite the sadness of this event I had to accept that pets don't stay with us forever, and eventually I had to move on with my life.

Later on in my final semester of school, I drew and painted a picture in art class of *Harry Potter* catching the golden snitch during a game of Quidditch. The teacher was very curious as to why none of the people of whom I drew in the picture had facial expressions. My answer was that I drew people that way because that was how I saw everyone in real life. This puzzled yet fascinated my teacher.

Another assessment I passed (even though it was outside of my main school) was my grading for Red Belt in Taekwondo. Red Belt is the rank prior to black belt, so it was quite a challenging grading. I was required to learn two new patterns, basic Korean terminology and to break a wooden board with a front kick. Board breaking doesn't generally hurt, however a bruise or graze can come up afterward if the strike is angled incorrectly.

Also, it must not be forgotten that as I was ending my time at school, Dylan had started Grade One that year at Calamvale Special School. He was lucky enough to get a place there (even though it was a struggle) because he does have Intellectual Impairment in addition to his autism. In order to be enrolled at that school, students are required to have an intellectual disability (where the IQ is below 70). At that time there were no publicly funded schools in our local city which specifically catered for the needs of autistic students.

His (and later Kylie's) school was a much better option than a mainstream school would have been for him. The teachers are specifically trained to teach students with his disability, the classes are very small, and the kids are additionally treated to fun activities that mainstream school students don't get (regardless of whether mainstream school students have disabilities or not).

CHAPTER EIGHTEEN

My family and I are in no way unsupportive of inclusion for all students in mainstream schools. In truth we firmly believe that every child has an equal right to be treated well and to obtain a good education at any school of their choice. Yet the sickening truth was that mainstream schools (especially those local to us back in 2007) didn't treat every student equally, and that gave me clinical depression and nervous breakdowns. Therefore our parents and I did not want my younger siblings to go through the exact same experience as I myself had done.

It could rightfully be said that putting our children into schools which solely cater for students with disabilities is not supporting inclusion. The need for an extensive change in our education system is so very important, and it's absolutely essential for us to fight for this. However our family (as well as many other families) firmly believe that we must not fight for this at the expense of our children's emotional well-being. In my own case I didn't enjoy having to emotionally and psychologically suffer for twelve years, whilst the education system made no improvements whatsoever throughout that long stretch of time.

At the time of Dylan's enrolment, Calamvale Special School was by far the best school for him. He made a large number of friends (both fellow students and even teachers), there were a lot of one-on-one lessons which enabled him to discover where his strengths are, and last but not least he had thirteen years of thorough enjoyment. They even got to have many fun excursions including a trip down to Canberra, to see the (federal) parliament house and the snow peaked mountains.

In my own school career I did have a fair number of very positive experiences; as I have shared with you in the previous twelve years of memories/chapters that you have now read. But there were still a large number of very painful experiences, including a memory from my very last day of school.

Throughout that year I was advised by my psychotherapist to use an iPod, in order for me to (solely) listen to some relaxation/classical music whilst at school. Whenever I'd be seen using my iPod (as they were normally banned at school) I'd explain that my doctor said that I needed it for relaxation music only, and would then show the teacher the note. Usually that was then accepted by the teacher or staff member.

Yet on my final day of school, when I was waiting outside the admin building for my mother to pick me up at the end of the school day, a teacher saw me wearing my headphones. I began to explain my reason and I showed her the note. But she said that she was not willing to accept it and queried as to why I was waiting outside admin and not the senior school carpark. I then told her that I was unable to drive, and that I'd been told by both mum and my support teacher to wait outside the admin building. Though she refused to believe a word that I told her.

After that, she asked me if I was intoxicated by alcohol or drugs because I had trouble maintaining eye contact (due to my autism), and that tends to give me a very blank and glazed look at all times. Then she took me to sick bay and told the staff member there to check me over.

I felt so angry and hurt (just as I had felt with that teacher I mentioned earlier from Grade One) because I've never even dreamed about considering the idea of using illicit substances. To this day I am still frightened to drink alcohol, and it even took a lot of coaxing to enable me to feel completely safe about using prescription medication.

Luckily though, the staff member at the sick bay was always very kind to me, and was appalled by how this teacher had treated me. Though once mum picked me up about fifteen minutes afterward, school was a chapter of my life that had suddenly ended. It was a very strange feeling. To describe it, I would call it an abrupt mixture of excitement, sadness and uncertainty.

For the remainder of that afternoon and night, I (like the rest of my family) was preparing for Mum and Brent's wedding, which happened the very next day. This was a positive distraction from my feelings about school. It was held at the same Anglican church that Brent's parents attended every week, and where Brent's mother taught Sunday school. The church was at Coolangatta, which is on the far southern side of the Gold Coast, and a 45 minute drive from our house. We had to do several trips back and forth to transport all of the decorations for the event. Thus much of the day was spent on the road, and much of the night was spent by us setting up the reception hall.

The wedding next day, on Saturday November the 3rd was very enjoyable, and afterward we had a heap of delicious cakes from Roberto's Cheesecakes. My personal favourite cake is their Black Forest Gateau, with the Chocolate Mud Cake being a fairly close second. Though I can never stand the taste of Pavlova or anything with coffee in it. We also bought a full-size 1920s style popcorn vendor (a modern replica which was powered by electricity) from a local store which sold electronics. It was used by us for a couple of years afterward, but it was always a nuisance for us to constantly have to clean out. So we ended up giving it away to some people who truly appreciated it.

Three weeks later Mum and Brent had their honeymoon, which was a trip to New Zealand where Brent could introduce our mother to his relatives over there. Kylie, Brendan and Dylan stayed at their grandparents' house for two weeks, while Jessica and I stayed at home. Yet our parents didn't want us to be bored whilst they were away having fun.

So they provided us all with a gift that could make us almost feel like we were on a vacation too. Mine was a DVD of the *Harry Potter and the Order of the Phoenix* film that had just been released. They also brought us a gift back home from New Zealand, as they were so kind. Mine was a 19th Century antique door key, as they knew that I had a liking for antiques. This is an interest I am proud to say that I share with my mother. I vaguely feel that my interests are equally genetic as they are environmental. Yet as for whether or not this is completely true, I will probably never end up knowing.

The end of 2007 was the completion of what was then the largest chapter of my life (school). But there were so many positive family events in November/December of that year, which made this time of ending enjoyable. The following year would feel very strange, and very out-of-routine for me. Yet all I would have to do was create my own personalised school experience, by doing lessons at home.

CHAPTER NINETEEN

NOW I HAVE TO CREATE MY OWN LIFE PATH

December the 11th, 2007 was when I came of age. On that day my family bought me an Xbox 360 console, which was the latest Xbox at that time. I also got a Nintendo DS portable video game console. For each of those consoles I was given three games, which did of course include *Harry Potter* ones. Then in the evening we went to our local all-you-can-eat pizza restaurant.

After eating there we decided that it wasn't really our type of place, but we eventually came back home to have some birthday cake; which was perhaps unsurprisingly decorated with an image from a *Harry Potter* film (*The Prisoner of Azkaban*, to be exact).

For Christmas I was given the *Harry Potter and the Order of the Phoenix* Xbox game, a few more Nintendo DS games, and my first ever Lego set which was a *Harry Potter* castle. I had of course played with basic Lego bricks during my childhood. But the 'proper' Lego sets blew my mind. It's not a lame and simple child's toy at all. There are so many detailed Lego bricks available that literally anything can be built with them. From that moment on, Lego became one of my greatest interests. Though nowadays I try to do as much digital building as possible, due to my guilt of purchasing a whole heap of new plastic which is so harmful to the planet that I love. However I'm very pleased that toy brick companies are currently starting to use recycled plastic in their products.

So with all of my new games and new Lego castle to keep me occupied, the remainder of December and the beginning of January was a rather productive time. I was entertained at the very least.

But the strangest thing about January 2008 was of course the fact that I wasn't going back to school. On January the 28th, all four of my younger siblings returned to school, but I stayed at home. Initially it felt a lot like being absent or even truanting. However it felt less so when I realised that this was the case day after day.

I received no qualifications or work experience from school, which meant that my chances of getting employed were very slim. As well, I was experiencing extreme anxiety and daily autistic meltdowns.

Yet despite all that, I wasn't considered to have high support needs in the workplace merely because my IQ is above 70 (in a cognitive assessment test I was given an overall score of 121). So I was ineligible to work in a supported environment, and at that time places that were specifically designed for autistic employees weren't even heard of, in the sleepy town where we live.

Therefore my sole income was from the Disability Support Pension. It's also fair for me to add here that I'm very lucky that I was acknowledged as needing a pension. I know a fair few people who have a life-affecting learning disability (such as severe dyslexia, in the case of Brent), and they don't even qualify for this support.

At that time, it did make a nice change to be away from the pressure of school and assessments. But I still acknowledged that I was then an adult, life was too short and it was only possible for me to live my life once. Thus the mere thought of not doing anything and throwing away opportunities was worse than having a year full of nightmares.

So I would use the hours that I previously used for school (school adjusts our body clock that way) to catch up on everything that I missed during those years.

In other words, I was essentially continuing school by doing lessons of my own. Throughout my days I would play educational games on my Nintendo DS (this was before I had an iPad), study the process of playing a chess game, learn about different cultures across the world, read about topics of science, and I would also practice/improve my writing skills. Many would ask me why I was so passionate about studying and doing all of this.

My answer was that it was highly unlikely that I would ever have a career. But I still wanted to use my time to discover where my interests are and learn all that was essential for me to know, just in case this ever *was* needed. Now I am so thankful I made that choice as it's enabled me to have less regret about that time of my life. Despite having struggled in my earlier years and having occasional worries about my future years, I'm very fortunate to have reached my thirties without a single regret in regards to my past actions. So all of that previous work was indeed worthwhile.

Also, for the purpose of preventing me from spending all of my time in the house (driving a car is an impossibility for me, due to a combination of certain cognitive difficulties and my medication), I would do an outing with my mother each and every Friday. The places we would visit were the mall, the antique shop, the local historical village, the cinema and the Gold Coast theme parks.

The purpose of these outings was due to my mum being concerned that I would otherwise choose to never leave the house, and would instead remain solely with my video games. This ended up working very well, and after a few years I was able to regularly go out during the week or weekend with support people, and not my mother.

Though in the meantime (in 2008) I would be growing accustomed to the process, by going to places I liked with a more familiar person. A few months into this weekly procedure, Kylie turned eleven on June the 13th.

It was a Friday, and while she was at school Mum and I visited Dreamworld. The *Big Brother* show (which we all liked) was being filmed yet again at that time. While we were in the *Big Brother* shop we were told that there were still tickets available for that night's Friday Night Live show. Mum immediately bought tickets for us all, as a surprise for Kylie that night. We ended up having a fabulous time and had Kylie's *Dora the Explorer* cake the next day at her grandparents' house.

As well, I must add something very interesting here. After the show we all got to meet the three hosts, one of them being Fitzy who is now a radio host (for the Nova station). Incredibly, many years later I ended up speaking with Fitzy a few times on his shows.

By extraordinary coincidence Fitzy (as well as everyone else who ran his show) invited me to speak about my life story on air with him, exactly ten years after the *Friday Night Live* show in 2008 (June the 13th, 2018). He told me that he could not recall seeing me all those years before, yet he agreed that the coincidence was incredible!

When you remember every day of your life, coincidences like these do show up surprisingly often. It really does show that our lives are indeed puzzles to ponder over and learn from. This book has been titled *My Life is a Puzzle* because it truly is, and every other individual person's life is a puzzle to work through also.

Skipping forward a few months I can certainly say that a lot happened during September of 2008. I was awarded my Provisional Black Belt after passing a Taekwondo grading, which we were all so happy about. Then in the latter half of the month, the house was all over the place for Dylan's seventh birthday on the 18th. This was because the whole kitchen was being renovated (sink, stove, cupboards and all).

However, after we'd spent all of that money, *typically for us*, a mere week later our hot water system broke! So we ended up having to replace that straight away too!

There are several times in our family's life when a heap of unfortunate events just get thrown towards us in one single hit. But then again, I must admit that there are many other moments when the exact same thing happens with fortunate events instead.

In the first half of 2009, I would receive a perfect example of this, with unexpected fortune that was to be very positive for me.

CHAPTER TWENTY

RECEIVING AN UNEXPECTED INHERITANCE AND MY BLACK BELT

On December the 11th, 2008 I got a pet cockatiel called Fawkes, who was named after Dumbledore's pet phoenix in the *Harry Potter* series. I also had a Tinker Bell birthday cake, as *Harry Potter* merchandise and cake decorations were very hard to find that year. We went to Sizzler for dinner and added Grandad's wife Diane to the celebration, who had her birthday on the 2nd of that month.

However this ended up being a fair bit of a hassle for us. In celebration of Diane's birthday the previous week, we bought her a rather expensive present and a nice card. Even though I was attached to that celebration (and it was my birthday on that actual day) Grandad completely forgot that it was also my birthday celebration, and he never once even said "Happy Birthday" to me that night.

I wasn't concerned about not being given a gift, though we felt that it was very rude of him to attend our event without any kind of verbal acknowledgment. Even when we sang 'Happy Birthday', he only mentioned Diane's name. Considering how much my birthday means to me, I felt extremely hurt despite being a grown adult. Afterward we made a firm decision that we would never make that mistake of joining birthday celebrations again.

The year 2009 began in a very similar way to the previous year. In late January Kylie, Brendan, Dylan and Jessica returned to school. Kylie began Grade Five and was having a lot of difficulty with coping. She had been struggling for a while, and it reached the point of her being assessed by the education department as being eligible to attend Calamvale Special School (alongside Dylan).

Mum has also reminded Kylie over the years that she was very fortunate to have had this opportunity. There was no way out for Jessica, Brendan and myself when we were struggling in an environment which wasn't geared up for our support needs.

In February of 2009 we bought yearly passes for Warner Brothers Movie World, Seaworld and Wet n Wild combined. We discovered when we returned to Movie World (having not visited for five years) that they still had the *Harry Potter* shop there. Back then there were no local pop culture stores that sold *Harry Potter* merchandise. Local stores in general didn't stock *Harry Potter* merchandise either, as the series wasn't as popular as it was previously; or as much as it would become again in a few years time. So the *Harry Potter* store at Movie World immediately became my favourite shop and I would always visit the park as a result of that.

Brendan turned ten on March the 9th of that year. His favourite interest has always been cars. So on March the 13th Brent had a day off work and took Brendan to the local race track, and because Brendan had turned 10 years of age he was eligible to have a ride in a V8 Supercar. Back in 2009 he only had a choice of Ford or Holden, of which he chose the latter. Grandad also gave him an authentic Holden Racing Team jersey as his birthday present, which he absolutely loved!

Easter Sunday was on April the 12th, and in addition to some chocolate I was given a Nintendo DS game which would teach me basic Japanese. Over the years I have continued to learn languages other than English whenever I can, because in this day and age it is more important than ever in an increasingly connected world. Currently I'm learning how to properly speak Spanish and French at a local tertiary education school.

Shortly after Easter both Jessica and I received a sudden shock. A friend of Jessica's was doing work experience at a solicitor's office when she came across an urgent notice for us both in The Courier Mail newspaper. This was extremely lucky as we didn't collect the newspaper back then, and if it weren't for Jessica's friend seeing the note we would certainly have missed this important notification.

At the time we initially had no idea as to why there would be such an urgent call for us in our state's main newspaper. This was well before the days when I did various media stories; and (even now) requests by journalists always come via email or occasionally by direct social media messages. But never are they so public and urgent as this 2009 notification was.

So we called the attached number and found out that our paternal grandmother had passed away and that she had left some money for Jessica and I in her will. We had not heard anything from that side of my family since I was ten years old. In fact from the age of six to ten, Jessica and I would only ever see our biological father every second Sunday. Though Jessica and I ended up getting a generous inheritance from Safta (which is Hebrew for nana, as she was originally from Israel), which we were very thankful for.

To this day I feel that it's very unfortunate (on the side of both the grandparent and the grandchild) that we never got to know Safta and became estranged from her whole family at such a young age. My final day of seeing her was when she came up from Sydney when I was five years old.

On that occasion Safta started teaching me some Hebrew. It's true that I didn't develop a close relationship with my paternal family, due to some very unfortunate circumstances. Yet as the family's language, culture and religion go back many centuries (even millennia), there are many generations of ancestors who contributed to my own genes and personality. Therefore I feel it's very important for me to learn how to speak and write fluent Hebrew in my lifetime, as the language is a part of my making. The same goes for Polish as well, as my mother's maternal grandfather's family fled Poland during the Holocaust to live in the UK. Sadly there would have been some relatives who were captured by Nazis and met a terrible fate.

Despite not practicing Judaism in worship, I do strongly associate the culture as being a very large part of my ancestry. Also, when I was a baby I was purposely given a Hebrew name, Rebecca, and that has various definitions in multiple regions.

From reading the story about me and Jessica receiving our inheritance from Safta, I felt this moment to be the right time to let you know a little about my family history on both of my biological parents' side. In regards to the inheritance, I have it set aside to use for unexpected and necessary travels, which are mainly visits to the University of California whenever I need to go over there.

On a somewhat bleaker note, in April of that year I injured my lower back while doing Taekwondo. As a result of that I had to take a couple of months off the sport, which really depressed me as I was determined to get my (full) black belt as soon as possible.

When I could eventually return to training in June, I was told to take it easy by my doctor because my back was still very stiff. This affected my turning kicks at first. However after months of hard and cautious training I finally received my black belt in September. To me, it felt like this was compensation for me not passing school. I felt so happy and proud of myself. This was primarily for me defying the odds, due to both my physical injury and slower than average processing skills from my disability. Those odds were defied by having my mind firmly set on a goal and refusing to give up. Even to this day I have to do this very often, and I must say that it does indeed work most of the time.

Later on in September, Dylan turned eight on the 18th and we had his celebration dinner at Sizzler. Grandad was there too and said at the end "that's good, all of this year's birthdays are over now". When he was told that I hadn't had mine yet, he said "well, all of the important birthdays are over". It was true that I was then grown up, but my family knows that my birthday still means a lot to me from very deep within. Also, when Jessica and I were Dylan's age and (in the case of Jessica) younger he had abandoned us, and never gave us a thought at all. So I was very hurt by that comment, and Brent assured me that he (without autism or an anxiety disorder) would have been upset if someone were to say that to him as well.

A few days later Grandad emigrated to Canada to live there with his new partner. Mum and Brent arranged a Sizzler breakfast, and later we sat with Grandad (and Diane) in the airport until 2pm, which was the time when they passed through to customs. We were assured that they had spent all night cleaning his house and packing up all of his possessions. Yet when Mum and Brent returned to his house they discovered that nothing had been done at all. The fridge was even full of food and his cupboards were still packed full of clothes. Brent and mum had been up since 4am but had no choice but to clean his house themselves. That took them until 10:30pm. Some friends kindly volunteered to help. I must add here too that he had been given the all clear by doctors to emigrate, and he was only aged in his mid sixties. This meant that he was fully capable of cleaning his own house before he left the country.

Late in 2009 we said goodbye to another (though much more pleasant) person who was relocating. My doctor and psychotherapist who I had been seeing for both counselling and medication, moved up to Rockhampton. The autistic meltdowns that I regularly experienced were still a problem, but my medication was stable at that time. He expressed to us that he felt it best that I try going without therapy for a while, and to just see how that worked. We did find that my medication requirements didn't change too much over the next few years, however it was eventually discovered that I would always need regular therapy for a combination of anxiety and meltdowns.

A little later on in 2009 we had our Taekwondo awards night on October the 31st. Given that it fell on Halloween that particular year, we were required to be in costume instead of uniform. So it was an opportunity for me to dress up in my *Harry Potter* robes.

Not only that, I was given another surprise that night. I had won the medal and trophy for Student of the Year! When I turned up that night I wasn't expecting any award, even one of the smaller category awards given before the overall prize. So me and my family were absolutely thrilled. It ended up being an even better night than I had expected, and I was so glad to have attended that event instead of bingeing on Halloween candy at home.

The following year, 2010 was set to be very similar to how 2009 was for me. Though it would be the final year of (what felt like) my time of confusion, monotony and numerous obstacles.

CHAPTER TWENTY-ONE

MY FINAL YEAR OF UNCERTAINTY

After graduating from school the previous November, Jessica turned 18 on January the 7th, 2010. She spent the night at Dracula's, which is a restaurant with a distinctly spooky theme. The place suited Jessica well as she's a quirky artist who draws and paints in that sort of style. Her clothes are inspired by 1920s–1940s Hollywood, and she has a liking of 19th and early 20th century silent films. Jessica also started university that year. I was of course very happy for her. But I couldn't help inwardly feeling very upset at the same time, because I myself was unable to get the required qualifications from school.

Unlike Jessica I wasn't eligible for an OP (Overall Position) score, which was needed at that time in Queensland to be able to get into university. However as several years have now passed, I've heard about several cases of special needs students entering university straight after leaving school (even people who were born in the same era as me). I'm quite confused about this as Mum and I were told by my high school that an OP was always required to enter university, and that being on a special education program meant that I was ineligible for an OP score. Since very recently I've began to question whether or not we were even told the truth by the school.

Throughout much of 2010 however, I still firmly believed what I was told by the school. It wasn't just my lack of an OP score or other kinds of credentials (needed for me to be employed anywhere) that were holding me back either. Due to being on strong anti-anxiety medication I was unable to drive a car, so therefore I was unable to leave the house without my parents. That too made the possibility of work or university a zero for me, unless my parents completely abandoned my four younger siblings who also had challenges, and their own work for our family's spray painting business. Due to my high anxiety and sensory processing disorder I was also unable to use public transport. During the days prior to the arrival of the NDIS (National Disability Insurance Scheme) it was very challenging for our own family and many other people who had disabilities. Even today it's still far from perfect. Unfortunately a significant number people (including Brent, Brendan and my sister Jessica) have been denied NDIS funding, despite having life affecting disabilities. Therefore I feel very privileged and grateful for the support I am being given, from both my loved ones and society as a whole. According to both my mother and myself I am a natural pessimist, and I have to constantly remind myself to look on the bright side and to also not feel sorry for myself all of the time.

Yet my life back then felt very much like a perpetual childhood and I was embarrassed to tell people that I didn't work, as a few people were accusing me of being lazy after hearing my confessions. I felt my life quickly slipping past me, believed I was failing and that I had nothing to look forward to. At that time my life seemed monotonous.

Though after saying all of that, I still had an inner determination to keep practicing skills that I was passionate about, just in case they were ever needed if I *did* end up working.

My career situation wasn't all that was on my mind that year however. There were indeed many happy moments as well. On Thursday April the 1st (three days before Easter) I saw the Dreamworks film *How to Train Your Dragon* at the cinema, in 3D. The graphics were excellent, which was a surprise because virtually every 3D film I had seen beforehand just looked like 'pop-up books' to me. After seeing that initial film I developed a liking for all of the following Dreamworks *Dragons* films, video games and TV episodes. It's fantastic how the main character and hero Hiccup has been made to have a physical disability. In the first film Hiccup lost one of his legs in a dragon battle, and another character named Gobber then made him a prosthetic leg. Gobber himself has a prosthetic arm and leg. Hiccup's dragon Toothless was missing a tail fin from the beginning of the story, and the film ends with Hiccup showing Toothless how much the two of them had in common. In the same way as the dragon needing a mechanical tail to fly with,

CHAPTER TWENTY-ONE

Hiccup soon needed an artificial leg to assist him with walking and riding.

Easter of 2010 was great too. Instead of heaps of chocolate I was given a pile of books instead, which included the *Guinness Book of Records* (2010) and some *How To Train Your Dragon* activity books. As a family we were given a few Wii games as well. Kylie's favourite was the game where the player got to create a baby, and nurture and care for the child until they became a toddler.

Kylie had her 13th birthday on June the 13th, and we had brunch at Jupiters (which is now called the Star), followed by a day's shopping at Pacific Fair. Then for the rest of the year I was planning for my own exciting celebration.

At the end of 2010 I had my 21st birthday. Luckily it fell on a Saturday that year, so I was able to have my party on the actual day. The weather was miserable, though I had a very enjoyable fancy dress party at home. Our garden was decorated with Christmas lights which looked beautiful behind the shimmering curtain of rain.

Little did I understand at the time that this was an exact visual representation of my actual life. By this I mean that what I experience in life is in truth happy and beautiful, even if those joyful 'fairy lights' appear to be distorted through raindrops at times. It is after all just a visual illusion, personal perspective and mind over matter. At that moment I had no idea about the changes that lay ahead for me, even though a lot of hard work would be needed to make positive use of those changes in my life. January 2011 was set to be the time when that long, slow and exciting journey would begin.

SECTION FOUR

A NEW DAY DAWNS

CHAPTER TWENTY-TWO

WELCOME TO THE NEXT PHASE OF LIFE

The rain continued pouring on down, day after day, week after week, non-stop for over two months (from late October 2010 to mid January 2011). So it was a cool, dark and bleak start to summer. Due to the bad weather we were unable to do our usual tour of the local Christmas lights on Christmas Eve. We were also unable to go out on Christmas Day. Yet with seven people living in the same house it's almost like a party every day. Mum braved driving in the heavy rain to go to our local supermarket, so that she could buy some Christmas food and fresh prawns. We ended up having one of the best Christmases we've ever had, as we didn't have to leave our home and we were kept entertained by our new gifts.

On Boxing Day my television (of which I had for a fair few years) broke. Though luckily Brent was already going out that day to get a television for Kylie, so I gave him a few hundred dollars to purchase one for myself. In addition to getting a new television, I was also able to buy an Xbox 360 Kinect with the $750 I handed to Brent. Boxing Day sales are an excellent occasion to find bargains!

The weather was extremely bad the next day. Thunderstorms came alongside the drenching rain we'd been having, and a small tornado even passed through our suburb. After the tornado we lost power and there were some houses that received significant damage. Luckily our own house wasn't damaged and our power was out for only 23 hours, as some other suburbs nearby had theirs out for two or three days. Though I used the time to put together all of the *Harry Potter* Lego sets I got for Christmas, including Hagrid's Hut and the Hogwarts Express train (which were the two largest sets). Once the sun had gone down

I did all of that work by candlelight. I've discovered that four candles light up our dining room table nicely.

It continued raining into January, and by then the ground had soaked in so much water that it could no longer take in any more. Our stormwater drains had also reached capacity, which says a lot as Brent had to climb down there once (several years earlier during a severe drought) to retrieve a radio-controlled car, and had seen just how big it was under the street. He told us that it was large enough and tall enough for a crowd of people to march through! However by that January the water was simply spilling out onto the streets and roads.

On January the 10th news had reached us that Gatton and other parts of the Lockyer Valley were experiencing severe flooding, and that the water had to flow down to the Brisbane River in order to empty into Moreton Bay. There were also fears that the wall of our city's main dam (Wivenhoe Dam) would collapse due to reaching double its capacity. Thus for safety reasons even more water had to be released into the Brisbane River. By that time all of our local rivers had already burst their banks and there was a lot of concern about how the king tide would affect the situation a few days later.

The next day all of the residents living by any of South East Queensland's rivers and/or on low lying ground were told to quickly gather up their valuables and move to safety. This included friends and family members of ours. The catastrophic floods did indeed come and caused billions of dollars worth of damage to South East Queensland, left many people homeless, and last but not least a fair few people had been killed. That was one of our worst floods in recorded history.

As January 2011 passed through, the wet weather slowly began to clear up for us, and more blue sky was beginning to appear at last. Similarly, the bleaker days of my own past were then beginning to clear also.

On Sunday the 23rd of that month I began the day by walking outside to feed my pet guinea pig. I was at the point of unscrewing her drink bottle when my parents called me inside to see something on television. Initially I asked if it could wait, but I was told that it couldn't be paused for a long time. So I rested my guinea pig's drink bottle on top of her hutch and walked inside.

It was a *60 Minutes* segment about a group of six people who had been identified as having a very rare kind of memory called HSAM (Highly Superior Autobiographical Memory). HSAM enabled those people to recall every day of their life since they were children in precise detail. Their recollections were being described as 'amazing' and 'incredible'.

I turned to my parents in a confused way and asked about why they were describing their memories as amazing, as I assumed that everyone remembered in this kind of way. They then said to me that it wasn't normal. Though I persisted by saying that it must be normal as even I myself could do it. That's when my parents told me that they believed that I had HSAM too.

Many a time people say to me "But surely there had to be a moment or two earlier on when you realised that your kind of memory wasn't normal". My response is always that me and everyone else who knew me were aware that I dwelled on past experiences more intensely than usual. Yet we put that all down to my Obsessive Compulsive Disorder, negative mindset and Post Traumatic Stress Disorder from my early childhood. Thus I truly and honestly felt that everyone was able to remember all of their life experiences; yet it was my belief that most people were able to cope with their difficulties better, due to them not having disorders.

In the previous sentence my negative mindset again presented itself when I assumed that no-one else but me has ever had problems to live with or experience. In truth, there is no such thing as one having a life which is 100% perfect and problem-free.

While I was processing all of this my mother asked me if it would be alright if she sent the University of California, Irvine an email expressing her belief that I had HSAM. The McGaugh and Stark lab at the UCI were the team who had identified the six people featured in the *60 Minutes* episode shown to me. I was half listening and said "Yeah that's fine". Though I was not at all expecting us to get a reply back. Firstly I knew we would be one of millions of people calling in, secondly I live a long way from California, and thirdly I'd never known us to be lucky people. Though after that email was sent all that we could do was to wait and see.

CHAPTER TWENTY-TWO

Two days later my younger siblings started their new school year. However early that morning a fuel tanker truck had rolled over and spilt a full container of petrol onto the local overpass. This barred us from using the Mt. Lindesay Highway, which is the only means of us getting anywhere. Thus the children in our suburb could not attend school that day, and the adults couldn't go to work. The truck driver who had spilt the fuel was at fault for speeding around a bend, and he was very embarrassed about the whole outcome (which was featured in the media) and he received a heavy fine!

Just over a week later, on the morning of Friday February the 4th I was due to have a haircut. Before I left I was watching rolling coverage of the news about Cyclone Yasi affecting places around Cairns. Then unexpectedly, Mum called out to me saying that the UCI had gotten back to us!

I went into the next room and discovered that they *were* interested in what Mum had said in her email, and they *were* interested in testing me to see if I had the kind of memory relevant to their research! A telephone interview was to be arranged for that, which would occur a couple of months after then.

Yet in the meantime (during March of that year) Brendan had been awarded a position of being an Earth Keeper at his school. This enabled him to receive a badge at a ceremony, and it was his job to help look after the school's worm farm, greenhouse and recycling plant. Roughly a decade prior to Brendan, Boronia Heights State School even taught me many important things about recycling, using cleaner energy, looking after our planet and gardening.

I also found it to be a very good school in regards to learning how to speak basic Indonesian, as well as participating in extracurricular activities. These included the multicultural group, which taught us a lot about all the different cultures, living on all six of the world's inhabited continents. Sadly many schools are now phasing out the importance of LOTE (Languages Other Than English) classes. Though today it's especially important to be multilingual, given that the world is quickly becoming more connected than ever before.

Thursday April the 14th was when I finally did my initial telephone call with the UCI. It was to be at 6am Brisbane time. When I woke up at 4:30 that morning my heart was racing and I was trembling in my bed. This was the first time the researchers had ever met me, and I had previously heard that hardly anyone passed the test. Waking up at such an early time, and getting my mind adjusted to 'wakeful mode' always means that there is no time for preparation. Also, with these memory tests we are told absolutely nothing about what we'll be tested on. So it is absolutely impossible for us to prepare ourselves; and to begin an assessment after having done zero amount of studying is *incredibly* scary!

Yet once I was doing the test I gradually felt more relaxed, because it wasn't as hard as I expected it to be. It's true that I couldn't answer questions about dates before I was born, though I was told that this was perfectly understandable.

However three quarters of the test related to events and dates from when I was alive, and also from when I had knowledge of the calendar dates. So I was still able to answer close to 75% of the questions given to me. A few hours later we were sent an email saying that I had done really well in the test. That was an enormous relief which elevated all of my cheery feelings for the remainder of that Thursday.

A few weeks later, Easter Sunday of 2011 was on April the 24th, which was the latest calendar date I've ever experienced Easter on. I was told at school that the first Sunday which falls on or after the first full moon (after the March equinox) is Easter Sunday. So it can fall on any date between March the 22nd and April the 25th. Each year the date can clash with various holidays and/or personal birthdays. For Australia and New Zealand ANZAC Day (April the 25th) fell on Easter Monday. Thus it worked out that our Easter long-weekend of 2011 was extended to Tuesday April the 26th.

A couple of weeks later, something quite different to Easter and chocolate had occurred. On Tuesday May the 3rd, we came across a baby blue tongue lizard who had been injured by a dog. We personally didn't feel it right to leave him outside in the cold to suffer. It is illegal to keep a wild animal as a pet, though we were legally able to nurse the lizard in our house until he was better, and then release him back into the wild.

Luckily we did have a small reptile terrarium and heat rock from when Jessica was planning on getting a pet bearded dragon. Sadly the blue-tongue did end up passing away as a result of his injury. Yet we were happy that he did at least end his life in relative comfort and warmth. As the lizard was dying, it was sad to see that he experienced a few tremors. This (kind of) links in to the 2011 memory that is discussed in the following paragraph.

In June of 2011 I had to have an EEG to examine whether or not I had epilepsy. This was because I was having various autistic meltdowns, and while I was having them I'd lose awareness of my surrounding environment. Yet the results of the test were that I didn't have any form of epilepsy. The truth was that while I was having meltdowns, I was experiencing so much anxiety that my mind would simply shut down and thrash around uncontrollably.

The results of this test gave me a mixture of feelings. It was a relief to hear that I didn't have epilepsy. However I also felt quite disappointed about yet another test failing to give me an answer, in regards to the severe meltdowns that I was experiencing...

Though on the other hand, July of that year was a happy time for me (and for virtually every other Potterhead) as the final film of the *Harry Potter* series (*The Deathly Hallows Part 2*) was released in cinemas. During the first week of that month I picked up some more Lego sets from our local shopping centre. They were The Forbidden Forest, The Knight Bus and another section of Hogwarts.

While we were at the shops we were told that the local cinema was hosting a midnight screening of *Harry Potter* and the *Deathly Hallows Part 2* on July the 13th, and there were still tickets available. As it was the final movie of that series I decided to buy tickets for it, and Brent (who is also a *Harry Potter* fan) came along with me.

We arrived at the cinema at 11pm and I even won the costume competition. I went dressed up as Hermione Granger, with her time turner and cat Crookshanks. Considering it was the early hours of the morning, it was incredible that the cinema was filled to capacity. Fans of all ages came along. Many of the younger Potterheads had a nap beforehand and were treated to a day off school the following morning.

The movie was fantastic and when we arrived home at 3:30am my mind was so full of excitement, as well as caffeine from energy drinks (which were cheaply and readily provided) that it took ages for me to finally fall asleep.

Later that month (on Sunday, July the 31st), Pottermore became available for a few people to use. Pottermore was an online site/encyclopaedia containing all the facts of the *Harry Potter* series, even information which was not included in the books or films. In order to win a position as a beta user, it required volunteers to be at their computer all day long, in order to wait for a question to pop up on the screen at an unknown time. Then the first few to provide a correct answer were awarded a beta position by the site.

However during that process I had a severe meltdown because I had been unable to do anything else but stare at a computer screen for eight hours, and our wifi was so slow that the question didn't appear until the answering session had closed 40 minutes previously.

There were going to be other questions like these on each day for the first week of August. Yet both myself and my family agreed that in my case it would be best for me to wait until it's public release a year later. The purpose of being a beta member was to help iron out all of the site's glitches. This would mean that I would almost certainly have had further meltdowns from time to time, if something didn't load correctly or acted in an unexpected way.

I did however have a positive *Harry Potter* experience on Saturday, August the 6th. Logan North Library was to host a muggle quidditch game against two local teams. Though as most members of those two teams were unavailable that day, this ended up being a session where all of us audience members were given a chance to learn how to play a simple game of muggle quidditch. I myself played as one of the beaters for Gryffindor. Also, it turned out that I wasn't considered to be as poor a player as I had expected!

After talking with fellow Potterheads that day, I felt that it would be great to join some *Harry Potter* fan groups on Facebook. So on Friday August the 26th I signed up for a Facebook account, and spent a lot of the next few weeks creating my entire profile and discovering the extensive world of early social media. At first, I liked exploring the areas of *Harry Potter*, autism, psychology, neuroscience and human memory...

During the days leading up to my 2011 overseas holiday, I spent a lot of time reading Jill Price's book called *The Woman who can't Forget*. Jill Price was the first person to ever be identified with HSAM, and this book describes her whole life story in regards to that.

From her earliest days Price had an unusual memory, and she can remember every day of her life since she was an adolescent, even though she has an exceptionally large amount of memories from her much younger years.

I greatly enjoyed reading *The Woman who Can't Forget* for a few main reasons. Firstly Jill Price's life story is somewhat similar to my own. Secondly both of us have never known life without having an excessive clutter of memories, and both of us experience much confusion when we try to comprehend the idea of not remembering phases of our life. Price described it so well when she explained how much confusion she felt when Alyssa Milano stated on television that she couldn't remember a whole filming experience from when she was eleven.

A year prior to finding out about HSAM, I myself got into a very agitated state when I heard my younger brother say that he couldn't remember a past flatmate who used to live at Brent's house. When my mother said that five year olds normally can't remember such early experiences, I disagreed with her and said that they would *have* to remember, because I believed that it was impossible to just lose a whole phase of one's life. This very confusing conversation ended with a meltdown, because I found the concept of forgetting a person who we saw every second weekend extremely difficult to understand.

Though, despite both Price and myself finding it odd that most people forget such surprising things, I previously didn't view this as anything worthy of deep thought. I just assumed that my inability to let go of things was due to my OCD. However unlike myself, Jill Price didn't look at her unusual memory as a medical disease, despite her struggling very much so with her inability to forget or let go of things. This was another personal reminder about how my natural disposition is to take a pessimistic viewpoint of any situation or experience (before thinking things over twice or thrice)

Jill Price knew that her memory ability was unique and wanted to find answers as to why it was that way. In the late 1990s to early 2000s HSAM wasn't heard of anywhere. Diagnoses of this condition plainly and simply didn't exist, as it was completely unknown to science.

So Price had to take the initiative by finding a research institute herself. One of the people she approached was a memory researcher with decades of experience from the UCI, Dr. James McGaugh. Luckily he was absolutely fascinated by her life experience, and was eager to gather together a team of researchers to study her memory. Price's courage and initiative to identify a characteristic of herself, do research as to how this could help her and other people, then to actively reach out to a professor she came across (expressing that she had a memory which science didn't know anything about) is so inspiring to me. There is absolutely no way that I would ever have had the courage to do that myself!

From the year 2000 Jill Price was given various kinds of tests, and then in the year 2006 she became the first person in the world to be identified with HSAM. Dr. James McGaugh also published an article about her case which (like her book) was named The Woman who can't Forget.

Jill Price inspired me to accept my memory as being what it is, and to involve myself in memory research studies to find answers (for myself, other people with HSAM and people with different memory related conditions).

Then (returning to my own life) October the 23rd of that year was when we flew off to the US for the very first time. This wasn't related to a UCI visit, but was instead a family holiday that we had been planning for over a year. We even had a limousine ride that morning. As our family owns a spray painting business, **Buddha's Motorcycle Spraypainting**, we're connected to a fair few local automotive companies. Thus we had a customer who owned a limousine company, and he said that for a paint job on his car he would arrange for us to have a stylish ride to the airport.

CHAPTER TWENTY-TWO

When we arrived at the airport however there was a small hiccup. Mum and Brent were absolutely certain that we would need a US visa, but our travel agent had assured us multiple times that we did not need a visa to enter the US. Therefore she did not arrange one for us, despite me and my parents being very skeptical. Though while we were getting checked in we (fully) discovered that what the travel agent told us was a heap of rubbish, and that we ourselves were indeed correct all the way along!

We were taken to another booth in the hope of applying for a visa (or ESTA) for each of us in the few hours we had left before our flight. With incredible luck they managed to come through just in time! It was so lucky that the day of our departure had to be a Sunday, as that was when the booth was open! Then they assisted us through customs, wished us a happy holiday and assured us that our (former) travel agent would get a very firm speaking to that afternoon.

Nowadays I know to have a Subway sandwich for breakfast before a morning flight, as it's both quicker to eat and can be wrapped up if I need to dash off somewhere. Yet back then I chose a bowl of nachos. It was lucky we were hungry enough to eat quickly (it was then 10am and we had been up since 4am) because barely 15 minutes into our meal we were called to the boarding gate!

This was also the first time that I had been on a 14 hour flight. Pillows and blankets were provided for each passenger, and we were told before the flight that the weather over the Pacific was excellent. So there was next to no turbulence throughout that whole air trip. That certainly wasn't the case with my other US to Australia flights. However back then I wasn't used to being sat in a vehicle for such a long time. Sleep is virtually impossible after leaving Brisbane in the morning.

During all of these flights hours and hours slowly pass... At first we fly forward in time towards an early sunset, cross the International Date Line and for the remaining three quarters of the journey the sky outside is pitch black. I think of this flight as a process of chasing the sun, for it to eventually meet us again at sunrise (of the previous day) at the other end.

A time always comes when I've watched all of the TV shows and movies that interest me, and I think to myself 'we must be nearly there now'. Yet that exact moment is always when I look at the map and see that we're only half way to our destination. So I then wearily think to myself 'we've got all of those hours again until we're finally there'. I also got bad airsickness on my first Australia-US flight in 2011. The reason for that was because my body wasn't used to such a long journey in a single vehicle.

Once we finally arrived in Los Angeles it was 6am on Sunday, October the 23rd. Australia is a day ahead of the US, so we arrived at the exact time and date when we left home in Brisbane (according to our different timezones). The biggest surprise for me initially was about how cold it was in late October/early November. Our seasons are the opposite in the southern hemisphere. Though despite being very tired we were excited about being in California for the first time in our life.

We had been awake and travelling for 26 hours, so the first thing we did when we arrived at our hotel suite was to take a nice long nap. I woke up at around 2pm to find my parents awake and my three younger siblings still asleep. Unfortunately though, I was very unwell with airsickness. It didn't cause me to vomit, yet I felt sharp intestinal pains that made standing up for too long unbearable.

But despite all of that I was still excited to visit Downtown Disney for the first time. It was true that my stomach was in agony whilst walking around. However believe it or not I did enjoy visiting Build a Bear and World of Disney. I even bought a dancing Tinker Bell toy/ornament and a Disneyland Resort T-shirt with Tinker Bell on it.

While we were traveling back to our hotel we came across a Denny's restaurant. Mum used to take Jessica and I to Denny's when I was three and four years old. Though all of the Denny's restaurants local to us closed down not too long after then. So that's where we decided to have dinner that night. I myself had a roast meal, and for dessert I had chocolate brownies and whipped cream. The US do the best of that, hence the reason for why I always have chocolate brownies and whipped cream there for dessert whenever possible.

When I woke up the following morning I was feeling slightly better, but my stomach was still too sore to do a lot of walking. However we visited Target after breakfast so that Kylie could buy a backpack to carry her things around Disneyland. There was plenty of Justin Bieber merchandise for sale and Kylie was a huge fan. So it's easy to guess what kind of backpack she bought. While Brendan was buying a new Xbox game, Mum went to look for some Converse walking shoes.

At Downtown Disney we met up with Grandad and Diane a few hours later, who had come down from Canada to see us. Disneyland is of course so big that it's impossible to see all of it in one day. However we did have a good look at Main Street and ToonTown.

By the next day my stomach felt perfectly normal again, yet there was a slight hiccup with my medication. Due to the differing time zone, I was having my night time medication during the day. This was making me very drowsy. We went to Disneyland first thing that morning and my mum gave me a Valium in addition, as a preventative.

We discovered that this was a bad idea when I was literally falling asleep every time I sat down anywhere! So from that moment on, while traveling I'll have my medication according to the time of day, rather than my own body clock. Also, I'll only take a Valium if I really need it (and not merely as a precaution) due to its strong side effects.

By the time the medication wore off I had a fabulous afternoon enjoying things like The Tiki Room, the story book canal ride and taking a train journey around the entire park. We ended our day at Disneyland by watching our first ever evening parade. Then we returned to our hotel to pack up our things for the next leg of that trip, which was Orlando in Florida.

As we were already seeing a lot of Disneyland on the trip (we would return to California again before going home) we decided not to visit Walt Disney World. Our trip to Florida was for the purpose of seeing The Wizarding World of Harry Potter at Universal Studios and the Kennedy Space Centre.

It takes a fair few hours to fly from Los Angeles to Orlando. However I was kept entertained by watching *Harry Potter* and the *Deathly Hallows Part 2* twice. By the time we arrived in Florida it was dinner time. We were taken to our hotel and thus had something to eat a couple of hours after we checked in.

At that time Kylie and Dylan liked Dora the Explorer and Go Diego Go. As we were staying in the Nickelodeon Hotel we got to have breakfast amongst Dora, Boots, Diego and Spongebob. After breakfast we went to Universal Studios to see the *Harry Potter* theme park.

In 2011 the park only contained Hogsmeade and Hogwarts Castle. Yet that didn't stop me at all from being absolutely mesmerised by the place. Virtually all of my holiday savings were spent in Dervish and Banges. My purchases included many things, including the complete set of Hogwarts house robes and all of the character wands then available (the wands were from Ollivanders wand shop).

I also paid a nice long visit to Honeydukes where I bought a chocolate frog, a Sugarquill and some Pumpkin Juice. We had lunch at The Three Broomsticks where I also had a Butterbeer.

The day after our first trip to The Wizarding World of Harry Potter (which was October the 29th) we visited The Kennedy Space Centre. That was the second place that I particularly wanted to see whilst I was in Florida. The KSC is certainly a very big place! There are extensive hectares of land with roads to drive through. Every so often we came across things like rocket launchpads, which look so much smaller in real life than they do on television.

When we reached the main exhibition centre we were absolutely amazed. There were replicas of the early space vehicles that we were able to sit in. Early space pioneers were correct by saying that it felt more like wearing the vehicles than riding in them!

After lunch we went on a tour through almost all of Cape Canaveral. We got to see the hangers of space shuttles, unused rockets (including a Saturn V rocket like the one that launched Apollo 11) and the control room used at the time of the manned lunar landings. At the very end we reached the souvenir shop which sold many interesting things that couldn't be bought elsewhere. I myself bought a pen in the shape of a space shuttle.

For Halloween that year we returned to *Harry Potter* world where I got dressed up in costume. I also made sure I purchased everything else that I wanted on my initial day, as I knew it would be a very long time until I returned.

CHAPTER TWENTY-TWO

After we left Orlando, we paid one last stop to California before flying back home. There we visited the Citadel outlet stores and Disneyland for the final time (of that 2011 trip). We also watched a medieval jousting tournament with Grandad and Diane. Then all too soon it was time for us to travel to the airport in order for us to board our flight back home to Brisbane.

Whenever we go on trips to the US we always board our flight towards Los Angeles in the morning. Though whenever we board our flight back home we always leave at midnight. That means we get more sleep on our returning flight to ease off some of the jet lag. I also didn't get unwell on this flight to Brisbane, because I had gotten used to flying by then. To this day I have never again experienced air sickness.

Once we had arrived in Brisbane it was breakfast time, and we had skipped from November the 7th to November the 9th (having crossed the International Date Line en route). We didn't need to eat breakfast at the airport because we had already eaten a lot during the flight.

After we had arrived back home, we were very tired indeed. Yet we still had to heave all of our luggage back into the house and our bedrooms. Sorting through our suitcases, and placing all of our possessions/purchases into drawers and shelves (as well as the laundry basket in the case of dirty clothes) is a very boring and miserable job. Though once we had done all of that we tried our best to go about our typical daily work. Going to bed wasn't an option as I needed to readjust my body clock.

Up until that year I had never before traveled far enough to experience jet lag. Yet little did I know that in the upcoming decade there would be several other long trips that I'd have to unexpectedly do.

CHAPTER TWENTY-THREE

NAVIGATING THE WORLD OF SOCIAL MEDIA

I turned 22 on December the 11th, 2011 and was given a Nintendo 3DS as a gift. Then two weeks later I received a new iPod, plus several accessories that I could use with it (a stand, headphones, external speakers and a cover). Personally I find Apple computer products preferable for me, as the easy-to-access icons and simpler layout give me less anxiety than Android/PC does. After all, the first computers I learned to use (at school) were Macs.

A short while later, on Sunday February the 12th we discovered that passes for the *Harry Potter* Exhibition down in Sydney were available for a cheaper price. In 2012 there were still no *Harry Potter* themed shops local to us; nor any pop culture stores nearby that sold *Harry Potter* merchandise. So we bought three passes immediately. I purchased my own, as did both Mum and Brent.

We ended up leaving for Sydney on Saturday, March the 10th (the day after Brendan's 13th birthday). Kylie, Brendan and Dylan were spending the weekend at their grandparents' house. Thus it was more convenient for us to depart from the Coolangatta Airport down on the Gold Coast, as Brent's parents' house was over an hour's drive from Brisbane Airport.

Coolangatta Airport is rather small and they've only recently started doing international flights. When we were there it was a one level building and there were no gates to board the planes. Instead we boarded the old fashioned way by walking out onto the tarmac and climbing a flight of steps.

Due to my autism I hated the noise and the smell of fumes. Though when I was seated in the plane I felt quite fine. The flight down to

Sydney was so much shorter than Brisbane to Los Angeles, as well as that of Los Angeles to Orlando. In fact by the time we were able to get out of our seats and walk around, it was barely thirty minutes until we began descending. The flying time from Brisbane to Sydney is just over one hour in total.

After landing we checked into our hotel in Darling Harbour, and then we had a good look around the city. Other than the rides to and from the airport we did all of our traveling around on foot (excluding a ferry ride past the Sydney Harbour Bridge and the Sydney Opera House). Sydney Harbour and the surrounding city look absolutely beautiful at nighttime. While we were out that night we did a tour of The Rocks and saw many historical sites around the area.

The next day was when we visited the *Harry Potter* Exhibition. It was fabulous there. During the tour we saw many genuine props from the films. There were also screaming Mandrakes to tangibly pull out of garden pots. Mandrakes are creatures from JK Rowling's wizarding world that are human-like plants with cries of which are "fatal to anyone who hears them". However those creatures themselves can be used to make a healing draught that can cure a person who has been petrified. In the *Harry Potter* and *Fantastic Beasts* series being petrified means to not quite be dead, but to still be completely non functioning; with the physical body frozen as if it were made of stone.

After the tour I bought some merchandise available at the shop. These included a packet of Bertie Botts Every Flavour Beans, an ornament of Harry's pet owl Hedwig hanging in her cage, a display of coins (a Galleon, a Sickle and a Knut), a booklet about the *Harry Potter* Exhibition and a book about the making of every single *Harry Potter* film that was released.

Once we had left the exhibition it was time for us to return back home. So we took a cab ride to the airport in the afternoon. While we were in the airport and on the plane I was still wearing part of my *Harry Potter* themed costume I went to the exhibition in. For that I had dressed up as my favourite female character, Luna Lovegood. While we were on the short flight back to the Gold Coast I started reading my new book about the making of the *Harry Potter* films.

The weather was stormy that evening in South East Queensland. Thus it wasn't an easy landing and we bounced a few times when hitting the runway. In our cabin some baggage even fell out of compartments that hadn't been locked properly.

Once we had left the airport, we collected Kylie, Brendan and Dylan from their grandparents' house, and then returned to the road to drive home.

After my visit to the *Harry Potter* Exhibition, my happy surprises in relation to this franchise were certainly not over. As mentioned earlier, Pottermore opened to a few lucky users on Sunday July the 31st, 2011. Yet it was in beta for quite a while due to a few technical issues that needed ironing out. I kept checking the site every day, and finally on Wednesday April the 11th, 2012 I saw that Pottermore were welcoming a few more people in.

So I quickly signed up for an account with all of my fingers crossed, and with amazing luck I was accepted in! The next day I spent the vast majority of my time on Pottermore. I enjoyed learning facts that weren't included in the *Harry Potter* films and books. Also, according to an expertly created personality quiz, I was matched with a black walnut and unicorn hair wand (rigid and 13 and a half inches). Then when I had done the Sorting quiz, I was sorted into the Hogwarts house of Ravenclaw. Prior to my sorting I was willing to accept whichever house I ended up being in. Though I was happy to be in the same house as Luna Lovegood, and also in one that was different from the two houses featured the most at that time. Those were Gryffindor and Slytherin (Harry Potter and Lord Voldemort's houses). In later Pottermore quizzes over the years, I discovered that my Ilvermorny house is Thunderbird and my patronus is a Basset Hound.

On Sunday April the 22nd I had my final *Harry Potter* themed experience for the year 2012. An Australian Pop Culture convention called Supanova was visiting the Gold Coast, and James and Oliver Phelps (who played as the Weasley twins in the *Harry Potter* films) were making an appearance there. So I went to Supanova to purchase my last few bits of *Harry Potter* merchandise, and of course I got a signed photograph of me with the twins.

Yet there were a few issues which held us up a little. It was hot and sticky the previous night. So everyone here at home was awake until the early hours of the morning. We had to leave for the Gold Coast only a short while later. Thus it took us longer than expected to get all packed up and ready to go. Also, once we had arrived at the convention centre, the machine initially had difficulties with processing our tickets.

When we finally entered the building, the crowds were jam-packed. Yet there were still 15 minutes to spare before the line up to meet the twins commenced. So Mum and I went to look at the merchandise available for purchase beforehand. I spotted a figure of Harry Potter with a (purposely created) wobbly head and decided to buy it.

Unfortunately though, the stalls were very close together and we had mistaken the shelf holding the figure as part of the neighbouring stall's merchandise. So I walked over to their counter to purchase the item. Yet the woman at the counter abruptly said that it wasn't theirs. A security guard (who had been barring our way forward) then led us to the correct stall next door where I wished to purchase the Harry Potter figure from. After that incident, as well as the woman at the entrance's irritabilities towards us from the machine not reading our tickets properly, I turned to Mum and said "they don't seem to like us very much today, do they"?

Though my meeting with the twins went much more nicely. We were held up while purchasing the Harry Potter figure, and as a result we ended up being at the very back of the queue. However I wasn't too bothered as I knew that I would still end up with their autograph, because I had already purchased it. There was also a somewhat unexpected privilege of being the last in line. By the time I reached the table where James and Oliver Phelps were sitting, there was no one else behind me. So as a result I got to have a nice long talk with them. They are incredibly kind people and they were asking me all about the *Harry Potter* park in Orlando, because they were due to go there themselves a few weeks later.

That same week however, I had an online experience that was no where near as good as that of Pottermore or Supanova. For several months I had been posting and commenting in a support group on

Facebook for older teenagers and adults with autism. I quite enjoyed that page. However a user who claimed to have autism selected me as a target. He repeatedly said that if ever he met or saw me out in public he would beat me to death, and that despite the group being based in the US he didn't live far from where I did (according to his profile he lived in Ipswich).

At that time I was very new to social media and had never faced anything like this before. Yet I ended up blocking him and I reported him to both the page and Facebook itself. Facebook dealt with the situation excellently, though the page I reported him to didn't.

The next morning the head admin of the page (I then ended up believing that she was possibly the man himself or vice versa) sent me a very abusive message saying that this man had been talking to her for a few weeks, and that he expressed to her that I was his partner and was treating him horribly. He had also said to her that my mother was orchestrating the whole issue, as she was "trying to break the two of us up".

With my mother's help (as I couldn't deal with something like this alone at the time) I expressed that I definitely wasn't his partner, and that this man's actions certainly weren't saying that he had a sexual interest in me; but were more rather extremely aggressive, life threatening and violent.

This admin however did not believe a word of what I said, and she believed that I was telling lies to hurt him and spitefully destroy his life.

Back then I could not deal with aggressive Facebook users like I can now. So I completely fell to pieces, and mum very kindly responded to the message on my behalf. When the woman accused my mother of profile hacking, mum explained to her that I had given permission for her to scribe for me in this particular case.

Mum was then told that 'non-aspies' (a slang term for people who don't have autism) are not worthy of telling an 'aspie' how they should and should not behave. That then put a stop to me ever posting, commenting and sharing her page ever again. I have had many experiences of getting belittled as a result of me being autistic or disabled (and a person doesn't have to be autistic to have life challenges/

disabilities). Thus I have no tolerance whatsoever for autistic people showing the same kind of arrogance towards those who don't have autism.

Nowadays whenever I experience online abuse I usually don't think much of it, and simply block and report the person without putting myself into a situation where they'll keep arguing back. Whenever a person harasses anyone online it's hardly any different to Siri verbalising taunts. Giving and receiving written messages via a computer is much less personal than face to face communication. So it's easier for cowards to taunt people by those means.

Yet in 2012 I had less experience with those kinds of situations, and felt that the way I was treated by that admin was very low indeed. I was extremely angry and my memories repeatedly dwelled on the death threats I was sent by that man, and the abuse and complete lack of care given to me by that page. This grudge lasted for two years, and then I finally moved on from it by acceptance.

That online experience really shook me up for a while, and I felt very nervous about talking with people (even to friends and family) on Facebook. Yet I knew that I had to continue using Facebook because it was helping me develop communication skills, and was therefore teaching me how to handle many of the challenges related to my autism.

For a long time I stopped posting and commenting on autism related pages, due to the experience I mentioned above. Instead I would visit pages about spiritual mindfulness.

Those pages ended up making me feel very comfortable, supported, and much more positive from reading the beautiful messages and quotes. I also made some very good friends through those pages. From me commenting and sharing quotes of my own that I had learned throughout my life, my friends told me that I too should start a spiritual page.

Spiritual mindfulness pages don't at all have to include mystical comments and topics. Sharing quotes by my favourite philosophers and historical figures also fall under the category of a spiritual page.

I was and still am very hesitant about discussing these topics openly, especially given that there are many people who think that my HSAM alone is very unusual (and some even claim it to be far-fetched). Yet both my family and therapists encourage me to be inspired by philosophical quotes, as well as to use Zen style meditation and mindfulness to ground my emotions into the present moment. So during the months following the incident on the autism page, I was able to feel much calmer and at peace with my emotions.

August 2012 was a great month for me. The McGaugh/Stark lab at the University of California, Irvine came back to us via an email. We were told that the reason for the delay was because it was discovered from their initial 2011 screening test, that various younger people (including myself) were considered to potentially have HSAM. Previously every participant in their research study was aged 40 years or over. So from the results of the 2011 tests they had to adjust their style of research and questions.

They concluded their email by saying that they were still very keen to give me further tests, and from the results of our previous talk they had me listed as a potential candidate for their research. Their testing would begin in the earlier months of the following year. Therefore the latter half of 2012 ran much more smoothly for me than the first half did. However I must say that all the media talk about the closure of that year being the end of the world really did irk and annoy me. Mention of this belief appeared to increasingly work its way into every single news story, as December approached.

Though at the beginning of December in 2012, a *Harry Potter* Spellbook game was released for PlayStation 3. It required that particular console and a PlayStation Move sensor/remote. At that time I didn't have either of those devices. So I bought them as a combined birthday and Christmas present for myself. The graphics were absolutely splendid for the era and I was thrilled to make frogs hop around my bedroom (on the television screen via augmented reality). I was also ecstatic that I could link it to my Pottermore account and use my actual wand that chose me via their personality quiz.

A week later, on Sunday December the 9th, 2012 we spent the day at our local water park, White Water World. It was a hot and muggy day. Yet my allergies gave me a very bad chest cough. I felt that it was just my luck to be bedridden and unwell on my birthday (which would be two days after then). However I was sort of lucky that I merely had a sore throat and stuffy nose by the time the 11th came along.

At that time, I had already been informed about most of what was coming up for me in 2013. This was because the UCI had told me and mum that there would be various kinds of tests in relation to my memory. However, the amount of intense work that would be involved prior to my HSAM diagnosis, was something that I hadn't previously given much thought to!

CHAPTER TWENTY-FOUR

GETTING DIAGNOSED WITH HIGHLY SUPERIOR AUTOBIOGRAPHICAL MEMORY

As usual, my two celebrations in December 2012 were very enjoyable. Perhaps my largest gift that I had received was a PlayStation Portable. Throughout the remainder of December and into January, I spent most of my time playing games on that device. Additionally I was enjoying my new Spellbook game that I purchased just beforehand as well.

Yet at the end of January 2013, Southeast Queensland once again experienced catastrophic flooding due to ex-Tropical Cyclone Oswald. With this particular flood event, more districts closer to our own home flooded in comparison to January 2011. On Monday, January the 28th we lost power just prior to lunchtime. Though I spent much of the daytime enjoying the cooler than average temperatures, and feeling the fresh breeze on my face whilst sitting outside undercover. Along with the heavy rain, the wind was howling and it is always a very peaceful sound to hear, especially at nighttime.

But it was lucky that our house was situated on higher ground, because we ourselves didn't have to deal with flood damage. Unfortunately there were many people in local districts who did experience those problems. Tropical Cyclone Oswald did make international news and there were comparisons to Hurricane Sandy given by a few journalists, as well as climate change activists including Al Gore.

But as was mentioned at the end of the previous chapter, there was a lot of work in store for me in 2013. Thus after the holiday season and the cyclone, it wasn't long until I had to focus my mind on what needed to be done.

CHAPTER TWENTY-FOUR

April of 2013 was when I began doing regular (online) tests with the McGaugh/Stark lab at the UCI. Due to all of its financial conveniences and greater quality, most of my tests with the lab from then on were done via Skype.

The time difference between Brisbane and California is a little difficult to work around. But for either UCI or media talks, I have still been happy about getting up in the early hours of the morning, as I know they are for a very important purpose.

Though I do still have to get dressed out of my pyjamas and look presentable, as the video calls are recorded; and in the middle of winter when the temperature from 3am–6am averages 3°C/37°F, that does take a fair bit of coaxing oneself! Yet luckily when I very first began doing these talks, it was a little bit warmer given that the season was autumn.

On Tuesday April the 9th I had my first (Skype) talk with the lab. I woke up and started getting dressed at 3am. My nerves were extremely high because I knew that the talk would commence in next to no time at all, and I had no other choice but to be completely unprepared.

Mum always gets up to support me during these tests by giving me a cup of tea and a plate of biscuits for comfort. However by the time I did that test, I was again surprised with how easy it was. I was asked about what day of the week certain dates fell on, and about whether there were any current affairs I came across on certain dates.

But even so, current affairs don't always provide clean cut answers for these tests, because most news events aren't just in the media for one day. People also come across news events at different times or perhaps not at all; depending on where they live in the world, and indeed whether or not they watched, heard or read the news at the time.

Though I was able to give a news event that happened anywhere within a week of each date asked. These included hearing the news of the disappearance of Madeline McCann on May the 4th (2007), the disappearance of Daniel Morcombe on December the 7th (2003), and the time when a man made a false confession of being Jonbenet Ramsey's killer on August the 7th (2006). After completing this test I was told via email that I did very well, which was a huge relief. But then, two Tuesdays later I was asked (via another early morning Skype talk) to describe in depth the emotional significance of those individual memories that I gave in the previous paragraph.

In the memory research tests conducted by the McGaugh/Stark lab, they don't want us to merely tell them the facts we know involving current affairs. Nor do they want to solely hear the day of the week for certain dates, as those are of course possible to learn and study at any time.

What they also want us to give them are the psychological details as to *why* we remembered those things, and how we felt emotionally at the time of those past events. The neuropsychologists researching HSAM know exactly what psychological characteristics they're looking for. Yet they won't disclose these to anybody, apart from fellow neuropsychologists or students working alongside them in the lab. Thus it's literally impossible to pass a HSAM research test, by faking or bluffing the answers.

Also during that month, there were (as always) many new media events occurring. Interestingly whenever I hear about news events (or remember certain news events), my mind tends to group bunches of dates and past media stories together. For example, on the morning of Tuesday, April the 16th (Brisbane is generally a day ahead of the US) I woke up to hear breaking news on the radio that bombs had been set off at the finishing line during the Boston Marathon. Throughout that day there was much speculation as to whether or not it was a terrorist attack, and it wasn't long until it was confirmed as being a terrorist attack. Yet, my mind was consequently taken back to the morning of Tuesday, April the 16th, (of the year 2007) when I woke up to hear news on the radio that there had been a campus shooting massacre at Virginia Tech.

My next UCI talk of 2013 was on the morning of Tuesday, May the 7th. For that test I was given three random years of my life, and then I had to explain my days in complete detail, from every date of the first week of May for each year.

The test took a lot of energy out of me, and out of tiredness I mixed up the year 2003 with 2004. Thus I had to begin the test all over again! So by the time I had completed the talk, the rest of my family were already out of bed and preparing the kitchen for breakfast. Of all the tests I've done over the years, I would have to select this one as the most intense. Though, there wasn't any time to dwell on that because exactly a week later I was set to have yet another talk with the UCI.

That would be on the morning of Saturday, May the 11th. Then I was due to watch a short video. The purpose for this test however, was for me to simply watch the video at that particular time, in order to create a memory for future reference. However there was a technical glitch with their video and it wouldn't read on my computer (and virtually every other research participant's computer also).

Yet those two hours of us attempting to get the program to load weren't at all a waste of time for me. In that time I had a nice long talk, and answered questions about the early morning sound of singing kookaburras, which was coming from the forest across the road from our house. The woman talking to me asked (as I live in Australia) whether I see many kangaroos around my local area. I answered that we do indeed see a few whenever we visit the local suburbs of Park Ridge and Greenbank. But unfortunately after us having this long chat about things, we just couldn't get the program to load; so the test was rescheduled for Saturday May the 18th.

In stark contrast, the video the lab wanted me to watch loaded with success that morning. This was the shortest test I ever did with them. All I had to do was watch a short film, and I was then told that I would be asked questions on a later date. That ended up being Saturday, August the 3rd, 2013.

However after completing and passing that bunch of tests in April and May of 2013, I finally received my official diagnosis of HSAM. That news was delivered to me via email, and I even got an attached certificate to print out as a memento.

Aside from UCI talks, many other events and changes were additionally happening for me in 2013.

After Jessica moved out of home earlier that year her bedroom (the largest in the house) was left empty. So it was decided that I should move into that room as I had a very large collection of *Harry Potter* memorabilia, and I needed more space to fit it all into. Kylie then moved into my previous bedroom, and Kylie's old bedroom (the smallest in the house) was left empty in case Jessica moved back home; as she did end up doing not too long afterward for understandable reasons.

It was August of that year when I moved all of my furniture and other possessions into the next room. This did mean that I had to leave my previous bedroom which was painted like Hogwarts castle. Yet my new bedroom got painted in blue and bronze, which are the colours of the Ravenclaw common room. Due to my autism I find change very difficult to cope with. So I arranged my furniture in exactly the same position as before. Then, as we rolled into September I had readjusted to my relatively new environment better than expected. Having cable TV in each of our bedrooms helped make this a lot easier for me as well. My new room was a lot bigger, so I was able to spread cushions around me and feel far more comfortable than I did previously. Then, a month later a new phase of my life began.

In October of 2013, I appeared in my first two media stories in regards to my HSAM. The first was in our local newspaper *The Albert and Logan* and the second was in the online *BPS (British Psychological Society) Digest Superweek*. This event featured a number of people (including myself) who had strange abilities, or 'superpowers' (as BPS described us as having). A day was dedicated to each one of us, and I was absolutely delighted about this. My parents excitedly shared my article around to everybody they came across!

Our articles were self-written, and mine was the very first blog post I had ever completed. Thus I was beyond happy when it got published on their site! That was later read by some other media sites and television shows, including *60 Minutes* Australia. From there further stories eventually came along later on, and doing regular media talks has remained a part of my life to this present day.

CHAPTER TWENTY-FIVE

UNEXPECTED SURPRISES

On my birthday in 2013 I was given replicas of each of Voldemort's horcruxes, from the *Harry Potter* books and films. These included Tom Riddle's diary, Slytherin's locket, the Peverall ring, Hufflepuff's cup and Ravenclaw's diadem. My family hid each of those gifts around the house, and then it was my job to search for them with clues written by mum on sheets of paper.

Christmas of 2013 wasn't at all my favourite that I'd ever had. The previous night we saw the local Christmas lights as a family like usual. So I went to bed in a very good mood and looked forward to the next day. Yet while I was asleep I had a bad dream that made me very depressed throughout the whole of the next day (which unluckily had to be Christmas Day).

I dreamt that I was a happy and promised young child. My parents had very high hopes for me, and they made sure that I grew up with as much happiness and opportunities as possible.

There was a day when my dream mother was dressing me up and styling my hair. While she was doing so, I was being told by all of the grown-ups in the room that I had incredible talents, and thus I would be enormously successful in my adult life.

Though eventually my childhood and adulthood slipped by. Then my dream parents and other family members passed away, and ended up long gone.

Last but not least, I did not live up to their previous expectations at all. The reason for that was that there were far too many obstacles in the way, which all seemed to come from my dream self's autism and anxiety disorders.

For years afterward I remained housebound at the place where I grew up, with everything rotting away before my eyes. I felt like I had wasted my whole entire life, disappointed all of whom had such positive hopes for me, and thus I fell into deep depression.

Eventually the dream house got fully destroyed by a fire, and I had to spend what little was left of my lifetime in a particularly horrible institution, of which there would most probably be none of that kind in the real world. In the dream everyone hated me at that miserable place. While I was being bullied I had a meltdown and then died from a head injury, because I became so old and frail in the dream. At the moment of my dream self's death everyone was so happy and relieved, and said "thank goodness we don't have to look after her anymore, she's God's problem now".

However my mind's creation of my actual mother then entered this dream, and she was sobbing as well as heartbroken, because she was anticipating the best for me while I was growing up. My mind also dreamt up all of the memories (those which actually occurred in my waking self's past) from when she was so hopeful and proud of me as a child. This made both me and the mum of my imagination sob even more.

Once again, I heard her say the words "I'm very disappointed in you Becky", and the distant memory of me saying as a two year old "Later disappointed, Mummy, later" flashed into the dream.

Immediately, I woke up in the early hours of the morning and I was devastated. It's extremely unusual for me to be affected so much by a nightmare. In fact I can (the vast majority of the time) control and change my dreams to go the way I want them to. Yet with that particular dream I was so emotionally/mentally absorbed into the situation and my waking fear, that it was pretty much like (unexpectedly and involuntary) coming across a disturbing news story.

Everything in this dream was a mash-up of all of my subconscious daily thoughts at the time. Deep down I felt like I wasn't the person who people hoped I would be as a child (due to my abilities being overestimated), house fires were always a strong fear, I was well into my twenties and still lived in my childhood home. The chances were also high that there would be no further generations to keep me company at the end of my life, and many had voiced to us that they couldn't look after me once our parents died.

For an hour after I woke up from it, I was still sobbing in bed. Outside of my emotional and psychological world, the dream wasn't of course real (in a physical sense at least). Yet, just as was the case in that nightmare, my life was indeed slipping by fast. Twenty four years was around a quarter (or more) of the elderly woman in the dream's life, and judging by how quickly that time went I would be her age before I knew it.

In the early hours of that Christmas morning, I felt like an absolutely failure; exactly the same as I felt shortly after I had been diagnosed with autism. When I thought about my life I knew I was disabled (which in truth isn't necessarily a bad thing), unable to live independently, was unemployed and had chronic depression with anxiety.

I strongly feared that I would end my life exactly like the woman in my dream did. Upsetting feelings and memories came along about me being denied senior qualifications at school. Also, in 2013 there was no government funding in employment services for the disabled.

So I then came to the conclusion that I was stuck with the life I had (with those imagined fears from the nightmare) whether I liked it or not. Initially, I viewed this all as negative because I felt that regardless of how much I tried, I was sure to end up exactly like that woman.

Yet it took a short while for me to realise that the woman in my dream was crying out of regret from the choices she had made, and also for what opportunities she herself decided to throw away. The old saying of "there are no victims, there are only volunteers" (which mum used to constantly say to me throughout my childhood and teenage years) does show its meaning in this situation.

Because, when I look back on my early life experiences so far (positive and negative) I constantly see that I've always tried to the best of my ability. So unlike the character who I was in that dream, I *don't* have all of those miserable regrets that she had. Also, I don't live in a world where every single person would view my death as a happy relief. Therefore it was so ungrateful of me to take my own subconscious fears of that seriously.

Failure itself isn't nearly as painful to think about as it is when a feeling of regret is added to the mix. It's indeed true that I never cry from feelings of guilt and regret when I relive memories of failing school; as I now know that there is no such thing as failure when a person has genuinely put in their best effort. In my most negative mindset the feelings I experience from those flashbacks, are twinges of annoyance (perhaps even anger) about disabilities not being understood within society.

It was unfortunate that I had to feel so depressed on Christmas Day of that year. However, unbeknownst to me that at that time, there was a pleasant surprise in store for me a few months after that event. But even so, prior to receiving that positive news, there were still some further moments of sadness to experience in the meantime.

Over the new year we had a severe heatwave in much of northeast Australia. On Saturday, January the 4th I came home (after spending the night at Brent's parents' house with my younger siblings) to find that my two pet guinea pigs had died of heatstroke.

Their names were Harry and Ron, and I hadn't had them as pets for a long period of time. So they were still young, but I'd known them enough to love each of their personalities. When I discovered that they had died in the place of their hutch where they slept I was very upset, as well as having feelings of immense sadness due to not having been home to take them inside the house.

That Saturday ended up being a 46°C/115°F day in my suburb with very high humidity, and as a result of all the events from that day I was both sweating and crying throughout. During that weekend I mostly kept to my bedroom and hobby shed. I also had a lot of difficulty whenever I was required to speak to someone. My natural tendency is to withdraw myself at times when I feel emotionally unwell.

Also, several of my plants and shrubs that I had spent a whole year growing died from the intense heat. So that added extra feelings of distress.

Though on a happier note, a week later on January the 23rd (which by coincidence was exactly three years after my parents showed me that life changing segment) we got an unexpected phone call from The *Woman's Day* magazine. We were told that they had received a notification from *60 Minutes* about my unique memory ability, and that they were very keen to publish a story about my case.

CHAPTER TWENTY-FIVE

This was originally planned for Friday February the 7th. Yet on that day the journalists had to unexpectedly travel to Bali. We were given many apologies (of which we completely understood) and the day of their arrival at our house was rescheduled for a later date.

It was very fortunate that I had that positive event to distract my mind, because there was soon to be yet another experience that I would find upsetting.

February of 2014 wasn't the happiest month for me, because a mere month after my guinea pigs had died, my young bearded dragon also unexpectedly died. His name was Horntail and he was suddenly getting tremors and having seizures. We took him to the local reptile vet and were told that he needed extra UV light and calcium supplements. I followed that advice and his tremors lessened.

Yet a week later I found him flopped on his back, semiconscious with his mouth gagging open. He was taken back to the vet, and later that night I received the news from them that he had passed away. Though the people who worked at Brisbane Birds and Exotics Veterinary Services were very kind, and they also made up a coffin with rosemary and a prayer attached free of charge.

However, on Tuesday March the 4th I received far more pleasant news. I had my regular haircut in the morning, and then when I came home I got a surprise phone call from the *Woman's Day* magazine. I was asked if it was okay for them to do an interview with me over the phone that afternoon, and then if it was fine for them to send a photographer and makeup artist to our house the following day.

Contrary to what many people believe, it's extremely rare that a person gets paid to appear in media stories, and nor do I ever expect money in return whenever I do these interviews. Yet the *Woman's Day* magazine did pay me for this interview, which was enough to buy myself a new MacBook Pro. I was delighted because it was the laptop I had desperately wanted for quite some time! My first story featured in their magazine was released in local newsagents on Monday, March the 31st.

Later on in March I also had some more Skype talks with the McGaugh/Stark lab. The first was on Tuesday, March the 25th and I was told a story about a pet, that I had to recall on a later date.

While we were on the topic I discussed the autumn heatwave we were having, and how I was keeping Hagrid (my new pet guinea pig) indoors all day.

My next talk with the lab was on Thursday March the 27th. Most of that talk was about me recalling lists of information I was given, and whenever another list was given to me I had to state which words were old (from the previous list) and which ones were new. Finally I had my last of that series of tests on Saturday, March the 29th. There I was told a story of a (fictional) gun shooting at the UCI, of which I had to recall later on. But most of that Skype session involved me being given kinds of tests that I had never done before in my life, though I ended up learning so much more about myself from them.

Firstly after many years of speculating it, I got firm validation that my photographical memory was not at all out of the ordinary. I was shown various pictures of black and white patterns for a few seconds, before having to recall precisely what I had seen. With that I expectedly failed, but I was reassured that the vast majority of my fellow HSAM research participants had performed just as poorly on that test as I did. HSAM only gives a person an exceptionally strong autobiographical memory, and autobiographical memories are just one of various kinds of recollections that people create throughout their lifetime.

On the other hand I found that I really enjoyed the tests where I had to memorise lists of words based on the colours given for each. As mentioned before, I had never been given a test in any way similar to that in my life. Yet I had then discovered that throughout my lifetime I had sometimes used the thought of different colours (along with smells and tastes), to help enable me to recall certain things in a quicker way. I was then told that many people who can remember a vast amount of their past (or lists of general information) have been found to have some form of **synaesthesia**, where different senses cross over and unite in this manner.

I had no idea at that time about what my upcoming UCI test would involve. Though in the meantime I had an unexpected event within my family, that took my mind off HSAM for a very brief while.

Easter of 2014 fell on April the 20th, and on that year we were each given a bag of magazines and/or activity books. However a few weeks earlier we had received some shocking and unsettling news, which gave us a feeling of not knowing what to do for almost a week afterward.

My grandfather in Canada had suffered a major stroke, and even though he survived there was still considerable brain damage and health concerns. So Mum and Brent went over to Canada to see him, while me and my younger siblings stayed at Brent's parents' house (of whom we looked after and kept company whilst we were there). Jessica stayed at home, yet I didn't as two people living together with severe anxiety is hardly ever smooth, for either one of us.

While we were down there we visited the local shopping centre often, and I bought a heap of new *Disney Infinity* characters and power discs. We also bought Easter eggs and chocolate bunnies. When mum and Brent came home from their trip they showered us with souvenirs from Canada; as well as California because virtually all flights from Brisbane to North America have to first stop by in Los Angeles (and perhaps Hawaii or other parts of the US west coast).

Two weeks after everyone was settled in at home we received some further unexpected news. I woke up at 6am to hear my parents in a deep conversation with each other. The subject of their conversation wasn't initially clear, so I had a hopeful thought of perhaps getting an hour more of sleep, as I hadn't slept too well the previous night. However as my parents' conversation involved so much talking and communicating, I had instead decided to abandon my thoughts of more sleep and to begin my day. Initially I didn't expect it to be anything out of the ordinary.

Though as I was walking towards the kitchen for breakfast my mother turned towards me, and said that they had just been having a conversation about an email that had arrived. My business email can be accessed by either one of us, and Mum said that an important notification had appeared in my inbox only a couple of hours earlier.

The memory research lab at the UCI wanted to perform an MRI on me, but that would require having to travel over there in person. Their funding was of course limited, yet I knew how important this would be for confirmation and credibility purposes. So I decided to use some of the inheritance money (that I was given by Safta) to pay for mum and myself to go over to the US for a week in July.

The morning we departed was on Sunday, July the 6th. As was the case with my 2011 holiday, our flight left Brisbane at just after 10am. We always have to arrive at the airport a few hours earlier, so consequently we had our breakfast there. Though unlike my 2011 holiday (when it was late October) it was still dark when we arrived at Brisbane Airport, and it was very cold when we stepped outside of the car. In Winter Brisbane's days warm up rather pleasantly, yet our nights do often get below freezing, due to the general lack of clouds in the sky.

For breakfast I had a foot long sub from Subway, with every hot pepper I could find, as I absolutely love anything super spicy (preferably Carolina Reaper strength). Usually Subway restaurants aren't open at 6am. However those at airports do operate somewhat differently. After breakfast we said goodbye to Brent and began the process of going through customs.

Having been to the US once before, we were fully aware that we needed an updated ESTA. But that didn't make the process of going through customs any less stressful for me. Something unfortunate at that time in Australia was that there was only one box to tick on the customs form, for carrying *either* medications or illegal drugs. Owing to the fact that I take anti-anxiety medications (along with prescribed Valium for emergencies) we unfortunately had to tick that box! This caused the initial officer to become somewhat suspicious. But their boss who was attending the neighbouring line told us that he fully understood about me needing medication, as his daughter had both autism and anxiety disorders (like myself). After checking the doctor's notes that we had brought along, everything was then cheery and fine.

Unlike my previous trip, I then had an iPad, which I was able to take around with me. I couldn't of course use my 4G without receiving a huge bill, as we hadn't had enough preparation time beforehand to organise satellite data (internationally) for our mobile devices. So throughout my whole (2014) US trip I had my iPad on Aeroplane Mode, which enabled me to use the device on wifi only. Prior to boarding our flight I messaged my family and friends on Facebook to let them know I was due to depart, and that I would message them again when I had landed safely at the other end.

It was a 14 hour flight and by the end of it I was exhausted (having had no sleep at all). After leaving customs I didn't get a chance to log into the airport's wifi. Thus I decided to send the Facebook notification once we arrived in our motel. Stepping outside of the LAX in July was very different from the time I did so during my previous October/November trip. The air was very warm, which felt so unusual having just traveled from my home in Winter. At that moment south east Queensland was having record breaking cold weather and California was in a heatwave. So it was a very interesting contrast!

Upon arriving at our motel we discovered that we couldn't use their wifi for our iPads and iPhones, because it was having difficulties. This made us panic a bit, given that our loved ones would have to wait a few more hours to hear from us. We felt that this would worry them. Though as I hadn't had any sleep for nearly 30 hours my mind was then too tired and sluggish to see any other solutions. My intention was to lay down on the bed, calm myself, and attempt to think about how we should solve the internet problem.

However, I was so tired that I literally fell into a deep sleep the moment my head touched the pillow, shoes on and all.

When I awoke and checked the time I realised that I had slept solidly until 4pm (which was a good six and a half hours). I felt well rested but still very panicked about the probability of my family and friends at home being extremely worried about us. Though at that time my mind was rested enough to come up with the idea of trying to log into the wifi on my laptop. Mum doubted it would work, but I told her that an OSX device was different to an iOS device (which iPads and iPhones worked by in 2014). Still mum doubted it, but I felt that we had nothing at all to lose by trying.

To me and Mum's delight it did in fact work and I messaged my loved ones straight away! Mum then asked if she could borrow my laptop to talk to Brent for comfort reasons.

Brent then told us something very interesting. He said that both the wifi and television were not working back at home either, and that our whole suburb was 'blacked out' (without any wifi, television or electricity).

Though we quickly discovered that our two experiences were a mere coincidence, as everyone else staying in our motel had the same wifi issues as we did. Brent said that back at home everyone was very distressed as a result of that, and that it was a relief to them all that we had arrived in California safely. When we told Brent that we were annoyed by our wifi difficulties too, he jokingly and exasperatingly said the words "We're worse off than you are, because at least you're with Mickey Mouse…".

After informing our family and friends that we were safe and well, we walked from our motel to Downtown Disney. Luckily we were staying so close to the parks. I made a Build a Bear named Tiana (a name from Princess and the Frog), bought a new Disney shirt for myself and had a cold drink with some ice cream. Then we entered the Disneyland park and had a look at Mainstreet.

Unfortunately though, I was feeling a combination of intense emotions/over-stimulation inside, most of which I wasn't aware of and didn't understand (despite them being my own emotions). As a result of that I had a meltdown, and this embarrassed me a lot.

But the staff at the park were lovely and reassured me that they had seen many other autistic people having meltdowns in the park too. Also a little girl came up to me and asked if she could sing a Disney song of my choice to make me feel better. She saw my shirt with the movie *Frozen* featured on it and sang 'Let it Go' to me. I had heard that song many times, yet not with a voice anything like that of this sweet child. Her voice made me happy again, and both the young girl and the rest of her family said that we were meant to meet each other.

On the other hand, it wasn't too long until mum and I had a third challenge (after previously having had a problem with wifi and a meltdown).

A little later we got lost walking back to our hotel, as the shuttle had dropped us off in a different location from where we had been earlier. Despite me knowing where to go from there, it wasn't worth attempting to walk in that direction (without using Apple Maps on 4G) whilst we were so far from home. Mum was especially worried when I had made the suggestion of trying. However, it wasn't long until another Disney shuttle took us back to a more familiar location. Afterwards Mum did acknowledge that I was correct in knowing where to go, and assured me that she just felt more comfortable with solely using Apple Maps and shuttles, in an area that wasn't our home town.

It was then time for dinner and we found a diner named *Coco*s where spicy Mexican food (along with other kinds of food) were served. Also, the cafe had excellent wifi. Thus we had breakfast there every day.

On that weeklong trip we visited either Disneyland or the Disney California Adventure Park, after breakfast each day. We'd be there from first thing in the morning, right through until midnight, and we got to literally see everything within that brief week. Though we learned for our future trips that it was best to purchase a HopperPass, which enables us to visit both parks on the same day.

During the daytime, as I was walking through the parks, I would snack on pretzels coated with M&Ms, dole whips and milkshakes from Flo's Cafe in Radiator Springs (from the Disney Pixar film *Cars*). As a result of the park being so big, a large amount of constant walking is involved from breakfast time to midnight. That's when our bodies do strictly require more calories and carbohydrates to burn! In Radiator Springs, meet and greets were available for two characters, which were Lightning McQueen and Mater. While saying goodbye to Mater I high-fived his mirror, and he said that I had amazing style! As well, there was a moment in FantasyLand, when I was at the top of the *Alice in Wonderland* roller coaster and waved to the passing parade. To my incredible surprise and delight they saw and waved back to me!

We did do some other things too, such as shopping at the Citadel outlet stores. There I bought some DC shoes, Converse sneakers (featuring a rustic American flag) and an Adidas winter jacket.

As the main purpose of this trip was getting the MRI brain scan, we did of course visit the UCI. While I was getting into the machine I was asked to remove all metallic objects, including my earrings and glasses.

I was also asked if I was claustrophobic, which is a phobia I do have even though it isn't quite as severe as my intense fear of balloons is.

The reason for why they asked me was because I would be inside the machine for an hour. As they additionally wanted to see what my brain looked like whilst sleeping, I was allowed to doze off during the second half of the scanning time. Having traveled all that way to get my MRI, I decided that it was definitely worth the chance to face my fears. With underlying feelings of jet lag, it also wasn't difficult at all to fall asleep when I needed to.

Luckily, the computer screen that I got to look at while I was inside the scanner gave me an optical illusion of being in a place which was a lot more open. Also, I was continually reminded (both inside and outside of the machine) that I could press a button to eject myself at any time. Afterward, mum and the research team who were present were very proud that I successfully faced my fear. I was even given some cash to spend at Disneyland that evening.

All too soon it was time to return home and I was very sad to leave the place, even though deep down I enjoyed the thought of getting back into my regular daily routine.

On our final morning I was literally in tears at the diner, and I said to my mother "this was such a lovely trip and I don't want to go back to Australia…". The trip had been so good that I strongly feel that fate gave me a weeklong Christmas in July, to make up for the previous Christmas Day that had been ruined by that horrible dream.

Like our previous trip we took a midnight flight back to Australia. Though it worked out cheaper to first fly to Sydney and then take a connecting flight up to Brisbane. Once we arrived home I was tired, but thoroughly enjoyed handing my family their souvenirs, and seeing their delight whilst unwrapping them.

After coming home from that wonderful trip, I honestly didn't feel like anything else would make me so happy and excited. I clearly felt that nothing could be more positive, or even equally as positive as that surprise holiday. However by the end of the following year (2015) I would unexpectedly be proven wrong.

CHAPTER TWENTY-SIX

LITTLE DO I KNOW HOW MUCH MY LIFE WILL CHANGE

My 25th Birthday was on Thursday, December the 11th and it was a very hot and stormy day. That year my family gifted me an original 1920s portable gramophone with some 78 rpm records for it to play (78s are the kind which feel almost metallic and are approximately a century old, or more).

Christmas of 2014 was much more pleasant for me than that of the previous year. My gifts were a heap of new Lego sets to add to the Lego village I was (and still am) building out in my hobby shed. Then, when New Year's Day came along my wish for 2015 was to have as great a year as I had (overall) in 2014. At that particular moment though, I had serious doubts of this being a possibility.

The year started off in a relatively quiet fashion in comparison to the previous year. My goal at the beginning of 2015 was to work on promoting and spreading news about my book idea. Given that there were so many other people doing the exact same thing as me, the task surely was very difficult. But after doing some research I heard that beginning a Twitter account gives a person a small head start with getting their word out there.

So I began a Twitter account briefly describing my story of HSAM and autism in the bio. My initial assumption was that I'd be posting things about my book to anyone who listened, and that it would be a smaller account than my Facebook pages (which were themselves very small). Though to my complete and utter amazement I'd wake up each morning seeing that I'd gained 500 new followers overnight! I'd also be asked many questions about my hobbies, career and daily activities. So as a result of that I updated my Twitter account each day with tweets, pictures, videos and links which related to all of those things.

Over the following few months this was keeping me very busy, yet very productive at the same time.

Shortly after Brendan's 16th birthday (on Monday, March the 9th) we had a family discussion about an end of year cruise. We had never been on a cruise before, so we thought that we may as well see what it was like. As Brent and his family are from and/or living in New Zealand, we decided to do a cruise around that location. This would also be at the time of my birthday. I'd never previously had a birthday away from my home city (and especially in a different time zone), and that made me feel a little uneasy. Though at the same time another half of me was excited about how this would most probably be my best birthday that I had ever had. All I was required to do was to be brave enough to change my yearly routine.

However, prior to the arrival of December there would of course be several other family birthdays to celebrate.

Kylie turned 18 on Saturday, June the 13th. That year, I got her a Build a Bear, which was of the character Stuart from *Despicable Me* (and The Minions). I also put a heartbeat inside of him and dressed the toy in Minions overalls, from the collection that was available for purchase in the store.

Skipping forward a few months, it was then Dylan's 14th birthday on Friday, September the 18th. He had switched interests rapidly throughout his childhood. Yet in 2015 he developed an interest in Star Wars, which he has stayed with permanently ever since. It's good that Brent (Dylan's father) is also a huge Star Wars fan.

So Dylan's birthdays (and presents in general) from that year onwards have all had a Star Wars theme; in the same way as many of mine being *Harry Potter* themed each and every year.

In addition to it being Dylan's birthday, there was a Skype talk with the McGaugh/Stark lab scheduled for that morning. But it ended up having to be rescheduled for the following Friday morning, due to technical issues. In that test (on September the 25th) I was asked further questions about news stories I came across on or around certain dates. One of the questions was about November the 20th, 2005. My answer to that was that I walked past the television in the living room and caught a news segment about the US president holding two turkeys, named Marshmallow and Yam who were reported to not like the idea of becoming Thanksgiving dinner! Despite voicing that with humour, there was still a large part of me which felt very sad about this story.

Then, two weeks later something unexpected and very exciting came along. Just as was the case with the US trip (of July 2014), there was no way that I could have possibly seen this coming.

On Wednesday, October the 7th I did an online interview about HSAM and my ability to recite the *Harry Potter* books with Press Association. That I expected to be a small online story. Yet I was completely wrong. Little did I know at that time that worldwide media get their news stories from sources like PA. So the next day I had media contacting me through all my social media, phone, email, my family's email and even the phone number of our spraypainting business. It's amazing (and in certain situations very alarming) what information can be found by searching social media profiles and my lists of friends/connections!

When I woke up on that Thursday morning, I was told that *Good Morning Britain* wanted to do an interview with me, and they asked if both mum and I could be at Brisbane's Channel 10 studio (for a cross studio broadcast) in a mere few hours time!

Mum rushed out to get a quick haircut at the local salon and I was panicking like anything! Though we were simultaneously very excited. A cab took me and my family (living here at home) up to Mt Coot-tha, where all but one of our television stations are located.

Eventually we arrived at the studio, and our driver spoke to security about us needing to be there for an interview. They were initially very skeptical. Yet when they called the crew inside and were told that we *were* due there for an interview, they were very helpful and showed us around the place.

While we were in hair and makeup I met Georgina Lewis, who I had seen read the Channel 10 news throughout my childhood. She was very kind and told us that there was nothing at all to fear about talking to a camera. Throughout this section I've said the word 'we' and 'us' a lot because they specifically wanted this to be a mother and daughter interview, given that mum has been such a major part of my whole HSAM journey. She was after all the person who always got up at three o'clock in the morning during winter with me, to serve biscuits and tea that would ease my nerves before Skyped UCI tests.

Live television is absolutely terrifying for a person who's not had much experience with it. So I was extremely scared whilst waiting in the green room with the rest of my family for support. However it always ends before I know it, and afterwards I feel so delighted about it all. It is in truth just like being nervous prior to being called up on stage to do a speech, yet for all that adrenaline to soon transform into a happy rush of endorphins once I'm up there.

That day we also got a request from one of Australia's top live breakfast TV shows (*Sunrise*). On Friday, October the 9th I had an appointment with my therapist. However in the afternoon I was free to talk to a Channel 7 News reporter (Damien Hansen) and one of the cameramen, who was very kind and has filmed multiple stories featuring my story.

On that following Saturday (which was the next day) I did an interview for Channel 7 *News* with both Damien Hansen and Kendall Gilding. Part of this was done at home and the other half was done at Queen Street Mall in Brisbane city.

My interview with *Sunrise* aired on the morning of Tuesday, October the 13th. Just like I do with HSAM lab talks, I had to get out of bed and put on nice clothes in the early hours of the morning. Once again I felt as nervous as I did before my very first test with the UCI. A cab picked us up at 5am and drove us up to Mt Coot-tha for a cross studio live broadcast at the Channel 7 studio (in Brisbane).

The talk went quite well, but when I was asked to recite the first page of Chapter 7 of *Harry Potter and the Philosopher's Stone* (The Sorting Hat), I had mistaken the first page as being the first paragraph, as a result of me being so literal. So I stopped reciting the page at the first paragraph, and the interview was over before I could correct the error!

At first I felt so ashamed and embarrassed about it, but eventually I got over that feeling and the comments on social media were all positive. That was a huge relief for me.

The following couple of months rolled along quite peacefully. Then on Saturday, November the 28th I visited Supanova in Brisbane and met Matthew Lewis (who played as my favourite character Neville Longbottom). The moment I began reading the *Harry Potter* books in the year 1999, I connected with Neville as he reminded me of myself in various ways. In the *Harry Potter* series every person who meets Neville for the first time mistakes him as being an overly shy and timid personality. Though once people get to know him better they realise that this is not at all the case.

Later on in the day we saw a live stage interview/Q&A, where Matthew Lewis mentioned some behind-the-scenes stories of his role as Neville Longbottom. This included the time when his ear got unintentionally ruptured by Bellatrix Lestrange's wand, as he was poked during a scene of *Harry Potter and the Order of the Phoenix*.

This whole experience whilst I was at Supanova was one of the main contributors to my feelings of positivity, in the lead up towards my birthday and upcoming holiday.

CHAPTER TWENTY-SEVEN

LOSING TWO GRANDFATHERS FOR VERY DIFFERENT REASONS

Due to the fact that we would be away from home on December the 11th (of 2015), my family sang Happy Birthday to me and did my cake on December the 7th instead. We got up early the next morning to take a cab to the Brisbane Domestic Airport. This was so we could fly down to Sydney to board our cruise to New Zealand.

Once we had landed, Sydney harbour looked beautiful as usual, especially as evening fell. We were keenly excited about the idea of going on a cruise. But once we set sail, we fully realised that traveling onboard a cruise ship is nothing at all like a boring ferry ride or traveling in an aeroplane (as I was previously concerned about). On a cruise ship there is a massive amount of space, there are duty free shops onboard, multiple restaurants, pools to swim in, beautiful decor, classes to take, and much more.

Formal night was on December the 10th and for that event I bought some exclusive Burberry perfume which was at a very good price. The Burberry Brit perfume was at a good price too, and I bought some of that later on.

Early the next morning I was woken up by a knock on my door, a birthday greeting and a slice of chocolate mousse cake from the staff in the galley.

After travelling across the famously turbulent Tasman Sea for over two days (from December 8–December 11), we had finally reached Milford Sound in Southern New Zealand. So, I went outside and saw the beautiful misty fiords at Fiordland National Park. We sailed through the fiords, mountains and waterfalls for several hours. It's quite difficult to access that region and the ship's crew said that luck was on their side that day. During breakfast my family gave me my birthday presents. Then later on at dinner time, the restaurant we frequently visited sang Happy Birthday to me and I was given another slice of mousse cake. Afterwards I was so full of rich chocolate that I doubted whether I could eat anymore for the rest of my holiday, or even my lifetime!

The next day however proved me wrong. We docked at Dunedin and left the ship for the day. Brent's sister and brother-in-law lived there, so for a significant part of our excursion we caught up with them at a local shopping mall. Margaret (Brent's mother) was also there to see us, because her sister living in New Zealand was sadly in her final stages of pancreatic cancer.

No trip to Dunedin was complete without seeing the Cadbury factory. There we got to tour the factory that makes Cadbury's delicious chocolate, and we got showered with different chocolate bars as we entered each of the many exhibits. Also, there was a room where we got to fill a cup with as much chocolate (liquid and solid) as we liked, for the duration of that part of the tour.

However, as the rest of us were walking through the door to the next exhibit we heard our guide saying to a guest behind me "Sir. Sir, we're moving on now. You can't take anymore of that chocolate".

After looking back to see who was being (humorously) told off, we saw Brent trying to sneak in a second fill of his cup! Mum said that this was so typical of him! Yet the tour guide was just as impressed with his sneaky idea as the rest of us were, and therefore laughed it off with us. At the end of the tour we entered a place at the top of the factory where 1000kg of liquid chocolate would get poured out of a giant bucket from above. However, that chocolate obviously couldn't be eaten as we had been told that it was re-used on every single tour (over several years).

During the rest of our cruise we had more stopovers. A few days after Dunedin we visited Picton where we saw an old whaling museum and the reportedly haunted port. Once we had reached Auckland our holiday was wrapped up by meeting Brent's niece and her partner who were living there at the time. Auckland is a little larger than our home city, so a lot was available for us to do there. We did some shopping at a mall in the heart of the city, then finally ended our holiday by each playing a game of miniature golf at the airport, before flying back home to Brisbane.

By the time we returned home we all felt that it had been a very enjoyable experience, and it put us in a very pleasant mood for Christmas and New Year. For me though, it was an especially important life lesson. That holiday taught me that it isn't necessary to strictly make my birthdays the same each and every year, and that it is actually *more* enjoyable to always have different experiences. Nowadays I've found that I am able to enjoy my birthday without being obsessed about the day's weather having to be a particular kind. Nor does everyone else in the house need to talk about the same things (within my earshot) and do the same activities as previous birthdays of mine. That was understandably very difficult for the people around me. As well I've learned that I'm not required to have the exact same cake and daily meals each and every birthday, in order to continue enjoying the event throughout my lifetime.

For a long time I was terrified that changing my birthday routine would eventually make me unable to enjoy the event. Yet this family holiday taught me that the truth is a completely different story. Also, from having all of these enjoyable vacations at various times of the year, it's additionally taught me that my birthday isn't the only exciting event of my life that I have to live for. Previously, this fear was the main contributor to my obsession of making that short (once a year) day 'perfect' for me.

As well, I've noticed in life that we're often more likely to experience a certain situation if it relates to something of which we fear. For instance, whenever I have 'risked' using an elevator (as a person who's claustrophobic) I have frequently gotten myself stuck inside. There is also a family member of ours who has always been worried and very particular about her teeth. Though she recently developed a very rare disease where all of the teeth are rotting away from the inside. Dentists are telling this person that they have never seen a case which has been more unfortunate (or even equally unfortunate)!

Many a time we hear the phrase "it had to happen to them of all people". However perhaps circumstances like these are blessings in disguise. Maybe it's life's way of easing our fears, merely by showing us that if certain events *were* to happen, it doesn't mean that they're quite as frightening as we initially believed. So, there is always a solution and/or an important life lesson for us to learn from them.

The following year, 2016 was a rather busy time for me. In March I appeared in *Woman's Day Magazine* for a second time, and later that month I did an interview for another online media source which was news.com.au. Once that story was published I had media contacting me again, including *60 Minutes*. It was then when we heard that they were keen to start writing and filming my story! This news meant a lot to us, because after all it was the original *60 Minutes* story about HSAM (that we saw back in January 2011) which began this whole life journey for me.

Just over a week later I received some other unexpected news which at first seemed to be vastly unrelated, on the surface. Yet I later discovered that it was indeed a puzzle piece which successfully connected to another (albeit with a sad undertone).

Easter Sunday was on March the 27th that year which was a relaxing and enjoyable day for us. However we received an unsettling shock as soon as we all got out of bed on Easter Monday. Grandad's wife had unexpectedly passed away from a stroke which was very upsetting on its own. However this also meant that Grandad could no longer live in Canada, as his nominee had passed away.

By enormous coincidence, he himself had a massive stroke exactly two years beforehand. Luckily he survived, but the stroke caused immense damage to his brain. So due to his medical vulnerabilities he had to come and live with us. For that reason we would have to travel over to Canada to collect him the following month.

This caused a lot of stress because the money we had left after our recent holiday was rather small. But we had to scrape our money together somehow, as Grandad was a member of our family. It was however a blessing that the flights and accommodation were cheaper during that season, me and Jessica had our inheritance money, and we (by lucky chance) received some work from a few customers at our family business. For some very strange reason life has a way of giving us the money we need, at times when we truly *do* need it.

Yet there was something else which was a lucky coincidence, and this is the puzzle piece connection that I mentioned just above. We received another call from the *60 Minutes* producers the following week, and they were suggesting the possibility of doing filming with me in the latter half of April that year.

It was there when I informed them that we were due to visit Canada the following month. This included California as well because (as always) it was required for us to initially fly to Los Angeles, before taking a connecting flight up to Canada. Also, I must too mention here that I've often ended up in Los Angeles for various unrelated reasons. This is another puzzling story about my life.

Straight after hearing this news the producers from *60 Minutes* Australia found this very convenient, as they felt that it was a perfect opportunity for them to come along (separately) to film me at the UCI and at the brand new *Harry Potter* theme park at Universal Studios in Hollywood. They also wanted to feature my story alongside someone else who was being studied by the McGaugh/Stark lab around the same age as me (give or take a few years).

Shortly prior to my United States and Canada trip, I had my first ever seminar talk about autism and anxiety on Monday, April the 4th. My therapist arranged it all, and she told me that an unexpectedly large number of psychologists, students, carers and special education professionals were very keen to hear me speak. The talk was to go for one hour, and I had never done a presentation of that kind before. Thus I felt very excited and equally nervous at the same time.

I'd have to say that on the morning of my first seminar talk I once again felt the same nerves as I did before my first UCI talk, and also those of which I felt before my first live television appearance. At that early stage I always wrote scripts for my speeches, and I've since found that talking for an hour equates to around ten thousand words.

When I had arrived in the conference room, it was a shock to see just how many people were in the audience. I turned to my mother and said "This seems to be a very big event. There must be a fair few speakers giving talks today". Then Mum and my therapist (who was stood next to her) told me that I was the only speaker that afternoon, and that all of those people in the audience had come to only listen to *me!* My heart missed a beat and I gulped. All of these therapists, carers, providers and community members seemed to have had a lot of confidence in me. What would happen if I disappointed them and completely embarrassed myself?!

Once I got on stage the words of my script vanished from my mind. Inside I felt absolutely frantic and I had an intense desire to burst into tears and run away. Yet I knew how important this was for my long term goal of making a speaking career for myself. This had after all been my dream since I was a young teenager, which was prior to me even discovering that I had autism or HSAM.

So instead of fleeing I just made up my script on the spot, while keeping to the structured genre of the script. As I was talking I realised that it was just mind over matter, and I was pleasantly amazed that the audience wasn't at all bored with my talk. Many even said that listening to me for an hour was much more interesting than having to listen to most lecturers at university! I was truly surprised and delighted to hear those very kind words.

A lesson that I learned for future talks was that (especially for very long ones) scripts are unnecessary. What I have to do instead is organise talks into structured sections, and speak for a certain amount of time in each of them. It makes everything so much easier.

Later on in the month we departed for our 2016 overseas trip (on Friday, April the 22nd). For that trip Jessica came alongside myself, Mum and Brent. While we were in the car, traveling to the airport, I got out my iPad to tell my friends and family on Facebook that we were departing that morning. Straight away I noticed on my newsfeed that the pop star Prince had unexpectedly passed away. Mum was saddened to hear this news because she liked Prince's songs when he was at the height of his career in the 1980s.

Once we arrived at the airport we checked in our luggage, then me and Brent each bought a Subway roll to have for breakfast. Jessica being vegan at the time picked something up from elsewhere, and so did Mum because she's severely allergic to gluten (having celiac disease).

After breakfast I went into the newsagent to buy an activity book and some pens for the long flight. I ended up getting a ColorAlive book (of which I can make the pictures come to 'life' with an iPad app) and a packet of scented marker pens.

While I was in the newsagent the song by Prince 'Little Red Corvette' was playing as a tribute to the late pop singer. When I approached the counter the woman who served me said that she recognised my face from media I had appeared in. This both surprised and pleased me very much.

She asked me where I was travelling to that morning, and when I answered her question by saying that I was off to Los Angeles, she agreed that it was a very long journey from Brisbane. Just afterward she asked me if I had a reason for why I was travelling to Los Angeles that day (merely out of curiosity).

In answer I mentioned that there had been an unexpected death in my family and that we had to collect my grandfather from North America. Then, looking around to see if we were alone together in the newsagent, I dropped my voice and told her that there was another project that I was involved in which would be filmed in Los Angeles. Though due to confidentiality I couldn't tell her who was doing the filming. Yet I mentioned that it was due to be aired on television a few months later. The kind lady then said that she completely understood about me having to initially keep this a secret, and that she definitely would keep a look out for my story!

Once I had purchased all of my activity books, magazines and books to read we headed over to customs. I expected and braced myself to be pulled over for inspection because of my anxiety, as had happened on every previous occasion. Yet on this trip, I just got a normal body scan and baggage check; the kind of which people usually get. I was wondering if I either had less anxiety because it was no longer new to me, or if I had just been very unlucky the previous times.

As was the case with my previous two Brisbane to Los Angeles flights, I had no sleep at all throughout the journey. Going through border security again (upon arriving at the LAX) was long and tiring, and something happened which initially scared me but ended up giving me a feeling of delight. An officer took me aside and said that he wanted a word with me.

CHAPTER TWENTY-SEVEN

At first I was very frightened and my parents gripped my hand in support, as we braced ourselves for him suspecting me of some sort of crime. The people stood behind us (who we had been having a friendly conversation with whilst waiting in line for an hour), even reacted with empathy towards me. However the officer then gave me a kind smile and said "Don't be nervous at all! I just wanted to tell you how much I liked the story I saw of you on Fox news". I then gave an apologetic laugh and my family and I all thanked him very much.

Once we arrived at our hotel I sent a message to my friends and family on social media saying that I had arrived safely, and then we had a nice long sleep. I woke up at 4pm, feeling much more rested than I was at the moment when we had arrived.

This was Jessica's first trip to Los Angeles, so we decided to show her Hollywood Boulevard as she likes (very much so) the history of old films and movie stars. Once I was dressed and packed, I went on social media briefly to answer my friends' comments and replies. Then eventually, once everyone was ready, we travelled by an Uber to Hollywood. While we were on our way there Jessica commented on how much Los Angeles reminded her of the Gold Coast in Queensland. I'd never thought of that before, yet agreed that she was in fact correct.

As a result of our previous trip to Hollywood Boulevard in 2011 we weren't initially excited about visiting. Yet Jessica had never been before, so we went there purely for her sake. However the rest of us were pleasantly surprised about how great a time we had there on that second occasion. This taught us to never feel discouraged to try something twice, merely because our one and only experience of that was negative.

Jessica bought a heap of Sephora makeup (she tells us that the US Sephora is much better than the Australian one), and I bought a heap of *Harry Potter* merchandise from Hot Topic (the US equivalent of Zing in Australia/New Zealand).

We also took pictures by the Hollywood sign and visited the Madame Tussauds museum which they have there. Being a huge fan of old Hollywood films, Jessica was clearly in heaven while she was looking at highly realistic life-size wax figures of her favourite stars. The rest of us enjoyed the exhibit too. I took pictures of the figures of Judy Garland, Vivien Leigh, and Fred Astaire doing his famous foxtrot performance 'Cheek to Cheek' with Ginger Rogers (in the 1935 film *Top Hat*). Once we had returned to our hotel I shared all of those pictures with my friends on social media, which also included a picture of Daniel Radcliffe's star on the Hollywood walk of fame.

The next day was when we visited Harry Potter World at Universal Studios (in Hollywood) for the first time. As soon as we arrived there I recognised familiar sites from my 2011 holiday, though I also noticed many changes that had happened in the time since. The park was mainly decked out in the themes of *Harry Potter*, *Star Wars* and The Minions (from *Despicable Me*). I'm as obsessed with *Harry Potter* as Brent is with *Star Wars*, so we were all in a happy frame of mind. Kylie's obsession is The Minions, and that's obviously where I got her souvenir from, in addition to sending along a large number of pictures. Jessica is greatly interested in The Simpsons, so we spent a lot of time in that area of the park as well.

We also did the studio tour which was just as good as it was when I previously visited, except that there were a few small changes which included a gyrosphere from the *Jurassic World* film that I liked. I've always thoroughly enjoyed this tour because it includes traveling through places where parts of *Back To The Future* and the *Jurassic* movies were filmed. More is included too. It's just that my personal favourites are the two that I mentioned above.

However my absolute favourite part of the Universal Park was definitely *Harry Potter* world. Whenever I'm there, I literally cannot stop smiling. I bought a bunch of the character wands that weren't yet available five years previously, in 2011. Unfortunately they'd sold out of Fred Weasley's wand, but I was hopeful that I would be able to purchase his on another trip (this will be discussed later on in the 2018 chapter). Honeydukes is also a great place to visit, and that was where I bought sweets like Chocolate Frogs, Fizzing Wizzbees, Bertie Botts Every Flavour Beans, Pumpkin Juice and Cauldron Cakes. Afterward I liked having dinner in The Three Broomsticks.

Once we had eaten all that we could, it was time to return to our suites and prepare for another busy day. On the next morning I had chocolate brownies for breakfast, and then we set out to Universal Studios again. While I was at *Harry Potter* world on that day I picked up my second half of *Harry Potter* character wands that I needed, then I went on the Forbidden Journey thrill ride. Brent and Jessica urged mum and I to experience the ride and I agreed it was important, considering that I can't go overseas everyday.

We were assured that it wasn't scary. I kept my eyes open because I never want to miss anything (or any ride) of *Harry Potter* world. Though afterwards Brent saw how pale I looked and apologised for getting me to go on the ride. So he bought me a Butterbeer from The Three Broomsticks to make me feel better.

We didn't have dinner at The Three Broomsticks that evening. Instead we ate at Luigi's in *The Simpsons* area of the park, as it was then Jessica's turn to choose where we should eat.

For breakfast/lunch earlier in the day I had a giant Lard Lad's Donut. Yet by dinner time I had made enough room to fit in two slices of a standard sized pizza.

The next morning we were busy with the next leg of our 2016 trip. We had to be at the LAX early to board a flight to Seattle (then to board another flight to Victoria, in British Columbia). The turbulence on our way up to Seattle was severe. When we took off we were informed that the weather would be very good. Though within less than an hour we were literally bouncing in our seats, with drinks and luggage getting knocked down everywhere throughout the cabin. On that occasion we were seated closest to the tail of the aircraft, which is known to be the bumpiest and rockiest place to be.

There was a man in our cabin who was swearing loudly, and a young woman a few rows in front of me was screaming and sobbing. I myself was sitting there quietly, though I have to admit here that I still felt very uncomfortable and nervous.

Fears of flying into air pockets had been implemented in my mind, by memories of a sadistic person from my childhood making up tragic stories with gruesome details, in order to make me too scared to travel anywhere. As a seven year old I genuinely believed this person's story, of supposedly being the sole survivor of a plane crash with dead bodies, blood and fire surrounding him. This person had told me that the crash had occurred by the plane suddenly dropping out of the air like a stone; which is physically impossible as even paper planes must glide down, in order to descend. Though whenever I experience intense flashbacks, my emotions and intellectual understanding return to how they were at the time of the memory's creation. So in this case, I almost returned to being seven years of age, when I had a limited understanding of certain things myself and believed all that adults would tell me.

That's when I began to voice this uncomfortable flashback to mum. Yet before I completed my sentence, a few other passengers went into panic when the captain suddenly made an announcement through the PA. Initially many were expecting frightening news. However nervous passengers were relieved when they discovered that he was merely assuring us all that everything was okay, and apologising for the unexpected bad weather. He and the cabin crew also reassured us all that the uncommon amount of turbulence we had then experienced was as bad as it can possibly get; and (as we had just seen) it was still safe despite being very unnerving to many.

After seeing the fear on my face, some really kind people sitting in our row assured me that air turbulence is no more dangerous than a car tyre (safely) going over a pothole. The two young men also informed me that there is a greater need to be worried during a flight without turbulence, as it's an indication that the vehicle isn't working as it should do; especially whilst flying over a mountain range.

By enormous coincidence as well, they lived only 20 minutes away from where our house is! The reason they were in the US was because they were aircraft engineers. That wasn't the only time when we unexpectedly met local people on (domestic) US flights either.

There was another moment when we were on an internal US flight, where the chances of meeting someone from our local suburb were far less than 1%. However, one of Brent's customers came up to him on the plane, and they unexpectedly had a conversation with each other about some current and future paint jobs! Brent was probably less surprised than the customer, because throughout his lifetime he's had so many other occurrences that were similar to this. He's only recently discovered just how unusual all of those occurrences were!

After a brief stop in Seattle we took a connecting flight up to Victoria, British Columbia. That flight was barely half an hour and was in a tiny jet plane, which still travels at pretty much the same altitude as a regular aircraft. Though due to its size, every turn and movement could be felt to a greater level.

Whenever I'm in a aeroplane I take my plush Harry Potter (that I bought at Warner Brothers Movie World in 2009) with me for comfort. Our flight attendant saw him and thought that he was absolutely adorable! She even asked me if she could take a picture of him. That particular Harry Potter which I own (with proper robes and a tie sown on to him as well as metal glasses) was made and sold exclusively at our local theme park over a decade ago. Whenever I have taken him overseas with me, he has always gotten lots of attention from people. Even stern looking officers working in customs and border security have expressed just how adorable he is, whilst being x-rayed! They've even (jokingly of course) advised us to get him his own passport!

Victoria, British Columbia truly is a beautiful place. It reminded me a lot of the pretty towns we had recently visited in New Zealand. Many of the houses were beautiful looking buildings. They also had proper chimneys, and not the ugly metal funnels seen on the houses in our local suburb. No matter where we went in Victoria (on Vancouver Island), we saw plenty of forests and views of the sea. There were also many deer to spot here and there. While we were traveling in the car I managed to take a picture of one to add to my social media, which my family and friends at home adored.

While we were in Victoria we stayed in the same hotel that mum and Brent had stayed in during their 2014 trip to Canada. Though we spent a lot of time with Grandad's late wife's family as well. Fisherman's Wharf was a great place to take a ferry ride, have an ice cream and capture a video of some sea lions playing around in the water. That was another post on my social media feed which my friends at home absolutely loved.

In the main part of town we had a novelty horse and carriage ride, and to Brent's delight there was a chocolate shop there. They were giving out free samples of chocolate mixed with lavender. I love the smell of lavender, and even grow the plant in my garden. Though initially I was very skeptical about how good it would actually taste. Yet to my immense surprise it was delicious, and I decided to buy a bag of it to both eat and share.

On our last morning in Victoria we visited Mayfair Mall, so that we could buy a few things we wanted. I bought a pair of DC Comics Converse sneakers and a Hogwarts bath robe from the pop culture store. Afterwards we went to help Grandad pack for his return to Australia, and then went back to Mayfair Mall for lunch. While we had been away there was a fire in Toys r Us which was a result of an arson attack. Fireman, police and news crew were even outside!

However the food court was open again by the time that we had returned to the mall, and I had a chilli burger for lunch. That day's hard work made us all very hungry.

The next day was quite a hassle. We arrived at the airport first thing in the morning, but our flight down to Seattle was delayed. To make things even worse, once we had finally landed down there, Grandad's luggage had gone missing. Catastrophically, it was the very suitcase which held his late wife's ashes! There was of course a great deal of panic.

But it was then when we learned to fully appreciate the time taken to tag each and every bag with a barcode whenever we're checking in. From that the airport staff were able to know that his bag had left Victoria and had arrived in Seattle, though it had gotten stuck inside the carousel.

We obviously did miss our connecting flight down to Los Angeles. However we got put onto the next Delta flight and had our seats upgraded for no additional cost. Then after we had landed, the third leg of our trip had begun.

During our final few days in California we visited Disneyland, and *60 Minutes* (Australia) did filming for their first story about HSAM. For that, me and mum visited the McGaugh/Stark lab at the UCI where I met a young woman with HSAM like myself (Markie Pasternak), who has now become a good friend.

Before Markie and myself met, both of us were told how to walk up

CHAPTER TWENTY-SEVEN

and greet each other. We were to be filmed upon meeting. Both of us were very nervous to begin with. Yet as soon as Markie first asked me how far back my memories go, and my answer was that they go back to the month when I was born, I lost my nerves completely.

It's such a pleasant feeling to meet another person who thinks and feels in the same manner as ourselves. Whenever I talk about how I remember in such an unusual way the two reactions are almost always amazement or disbelief. Yet being able to speak to someone who views the situation as being a *normal* part of life, and who's able to participate with you in a light hearted/humorous conversation about all of the annoyances you each share, is a positive feeling which no other experience can compete with.

Many more questions were asked between us, including me asking Markie if she also looked at New Year as going back in time rather than going forward in time. Whenever it's New Year, I cannot help but notice the calendar winding all the way down from December the 31st to January the 1st (without considering that the year has moved upwards). We were both delighted when she answered 'yes' to that.

Markie and I kept on talking, which impressed the crew filming us very much. In fact most of our initial conversation was as natural as if the camera wasn't there. Once the recording had stopped, we kept on talking and even joked about how in years to come we would laugh about how we first met while we were being filmed by *60 Minutes*!

The filming at the UCI however did not end at that point. After Markie and I met, we went into the research lab and had some lunch at a Starbucks café. I don't like the taste of any kind of coffee (as it's far too bitter), but I absolutely love their spicy chai lattes without coffee. Here in Australia we have an enormous amount of Coffee Club cafés around, because the franchise is Australian. Though we do also have a large number of Starbucks cafés too, and that pleases me very much. As well, there are numerous other café chains available in Australia which are very good also. It's not a mere stereotype that most Australians love their coffees and frappes!

After lunch we were (separately) called into a room to answer a few memory related questions on film. Then we were individually filmed in the MRI machine. As I had done my MRI with the McGaugh/Stark lab in 2014, the one I did for the *60 Minutes* episode two years later was just of me laid down in the machine. Yet, it was the results from my 2014 MRI session which were talked over and included in the episode.

After leaving the UCI, Mum and I returned to our hotel where we met up with Brent, Grandad and Jessica. We had pizza for dinner and then visited Downtown Disney. Jessica spent most of her evening at Sephora, and I went to Build a Bear and the Lego Store. Build a Bear was very busy that night. Yet I made a (Disneyland) Diamond Celebration Bear and a limited edition Ariel Bear. Along with the bears, I bought a few scents to place inside of them (both for the bears I made that night, and for my unscented bears I already had at home). As well, I bought some new Disneyland clothes/accessories for my furry friends that I built, which weren't available on my previous trip. After Build a Bear we went to the Lego Store, where I bought a scaled down version of Big Ben for the London section of my Lego village.

Finally I met up with Brent, Jessica and Grandad outside a restaurant. By that time it was midnight. Despite being so tired I was still somewhat surprised about how late it actually was! Due to being in a rush after leaving the lab, returning to the hotel, having a hurried dinner and racing to get dressed/showered to go out, time seemed to have slipped by very quickly indeed.

As well, I only realised at midnight that I hadn't taken my anti-anxiety medication! As a result of my autism and OCD, I have to live my life in a set routine. I normally have my nighttime medication at 8:30pm, but I got distracted by the overload of other activities required of me at that time. This is one of many examples I give to people, whenever I'm queried as to whether it *truly* is the case that I cannot do multiple tasks simultaneously. The plain and simple truth is that I can't.

Just as I was set to take the pills kept in my bag, I additionally realised that I had already drank all of the water from my water bottle!

Thus my anxiety level was very high. But when I finally took my regular nighttime medication (after Brent ordered a jug of water), my mother also handed me a Valium tablet to take, and that calmed me down quite quickly. As Valium is very strong, our doctor's instructions have been for me to only to take one tablet at times when I strictly need it, and to never take more than one in a 24hr period.

Though I wasn't the only one who was worked up by the end of that evening. Grandad was being sulky and bad tempered that night, which was why mum was unable to initially meet up with us in Build a Bear. She had spent that evening telling Grandad to behave himself, as he kept arguing about wanting a scooter instead of a wheelchair. Though he was unable to have a scooter due to his 2014 stroke affecting his vision and motor skills. So mum had a very stressful and exhausting night.

The next day was Grandad's 75th birthday celebration, and we got up bright and early to spend the entire day at Disneyland, as he had always expressed how much he liked the park. Overall it was a very enjoyable day for me. Brent got to see Radiator Springs from *Cars* the Movie for the first time, and Jessica got to see the two Disney Parks themselves for the first time.

In Main Street I bought my Mickey ears for that trip, which featured the Mad Hatter from *Alice in Wonderland*. I also got my name 'Becky' embroidered on them. We then visited Adventureland and Frontierland to buy Grandad's birthday presents. In the evening we watched the parade in Main Street and spent our time until midnight exploring Fantasyland. I had a great time there and even found some new Disney charms to add to my bracelet (Mickey Mouse on *Steamboat Willie* and Tinkerbell).

There was also a plush toy of Sully holding Mike Wazowski which I liked and bought. However when I took him to the counter he seemed to struggle with getting into his bag. Mum jokingly said that it was as if he didn't want to travel all the way to Australia and wanted to stay at Disneyland for ever. I then looked at Sully and said "I know how you feel…". To this day I always make sure that he's out in the open in my bedroom and surrounded by Disneyland purchases, or at the very least with Disney merchandise bought from elsewhere.

The final day of our 2016 US trip was very busy indeed. I met up again with the *60 Minutes* crew at Universal Studios. There I did a short interview whilst walking through Hogsmeade, and I checked to see if they had gotten more Fred Weasley wands. Unfortunately they still hadn't ordered new ones in, so I had to put that wand on the list of purchases for my next trip there. However, I had already bought a sizeable number of new character wands during that trip anyway.

After Universal Studios we paid one last visit to the Disney Parks before returning home late that night. At California Adventure we watched the parade featuring the Disney Pixar characters, and that was very enjoyable. I did have a meltdown in a cafe due to being overstimulated with noise, and from being constantly rushed along that day. Yet a Valium tablet brought me back down quickly, despite leaving me with much embarrassment.

However, after going on my favourite ride in that park (*Monsters Inc. Mike and Sulley to the Rescue*) I was able to put those negative thoughts about an unchangeable issue behind me. Just as the old expression says "there's no use crying over spilt milk".

Finally when evening came it was time to go to the airport to take a flight back home. We were tired and exhausted, and were at the stage where the thought of returning home was pleasant; until a few months later when we'd be longing for another overseas trip.

Grandad however, wasn't too happy about traveling home in economy, and he couldn't see why they wouldn't upgrade his seat for free. At the check-in counter Brent then said "Go and ask them yourself and you'll hear the exact same answer that we're giving you". That he did, and he demanded a business class seat without success, despite the woman talking to him kindly.

In the departure lounge he was ranting about her not giving him his own way, and was sulking for hours (both in the lounge and on the plane). Mum and Brent explained to him that he was not capable of being on his own and needed our care. Grandad then yelled at them saying that he didn't like being treated like a 'mental retard'. Mum then said that if he was indeed acting like he was less competent than he really was, it made his behaviour over the past few days even worse. She also asked him to apologise on behalf of two of her own children who do have an Intellectual Disability, and that to refer to the disability they have in such a derogative manner was insulting.

CHAPTER TWENTY-SEVEN

Our flight was at midnight, though it takes around 20 minutes to reach the runway leading off to Brisbane. But I was so tired that I fell asleep before we even took off. I slipped into dreams about me being settled and back into routine at home. This made me feel so content. It's always nice to think about your own comfortable bed which isn't in a hotel suite...

However, a couple of sharp bumps brought the realisation to my mind that I was not yet at home, and I was still on a plane. By the time I woke up from this lucid dream, the whole cabin seemed to be asleep. I had no idea what time it was or where we were in our flight.

Though I asked my mother (who was then awake) when dinner was going to be served. Mum then said that dinner was served hours ago, but it looked to her like I was deeply asleep, and she didn't feel it right to wake me up from such a fortunate state. I wasn't hungry anyway, as I had eaten a lot of food when we were at Universal Studios and Disneyland.

Looking at the map showing the progress of our flight, I saw that we were more than half way home. This made me realise that I'd somehow managed to have a full cycle of sleep. After then however, I couldn't get back to sleep. Yet there weren't too many hours left before we landed anyhow.

We arrived back in Brisbane on the morning of May the 3rd, 2016. I was absolutely exhausted and felt (at that moment) like I was completely over traveling anywhere, and was glad to have arrived safely back home. Before taking a cab ride to our house I messaged my friends and family on Facebook, saying that everything was well. We ate our breakfast at the airport. Once I was back home however, I spent the whole day unpacking my suitcases and fighting the temptation to climb into bed and fall asleep.

A few weeks later (on Tuesday, May the 23rd) I visited The University of Queensland (UQ) who had expressed an interest in conducting a research study about my HSAM and autism. Puzzlingly, this had all come from my mother going to have a hearing test.

Due to a side-effect of the medication she was given in hospital for a 2002 operation, Mum had developed significant hearing loss in one of her ears. So after a test at a local clinic, it was revealed that she would have to wear a hearing aid. Consequently, Mum got a chance to speak about all of her (then) current goings on, as there was a significant amount of time needed to fully organise her prescription.

While Mum was talking about my HSAM tests at the UCI, and our thoughts of contacting the Queensland Brain Institute (at the University of Queensland) the audiologist told Mum that a close family member of hers worked with the people involved there, and that she would definitely pass on the information Mum gave to her.

In the exact same way as when we first contacted the UCI, I was amazed and delighted about how quick and positive the reply was. Incredibly, just like the McGaugh/Stark lab at the UCI, they too were very keen to study my case and the condition of HSAM itself!

I met up with Professor Gail Robinson who is conducting this research study, as well as one of her students, Emily Gibson who assisted her with research (later on in this book there will be other assisting students mentioned). They were both such lovely people, and they were delighted when I agreed to sign the contract for their study. After getting started with some initial tests (to see where my baseline was for future testing) it was 2pm by the time Mum and I got home. Over the next few weeks I had two more visits to UQ where further baseline tests were conducted.

During that time, further filming for *60 Minutes* was done of me at home. Footage that was included was of my *Harry Potter* memorabilia, the Lego village I've been building in my shed, me reciting chapters of *Harry Potter*, and also there was a clip of my mother and I making a cup of tea in the kitchen.

In contrast however, June and July in the year 2016 were very traumatic family wise. Brent's dad George had initially been admitted to hospital with a brain tumour. Given the fact that he was 87 years old, we had been told by the hospital that there was a strong likelihood of him not surviving the cancer itself, or the operation/treatment. When we saw him at Tweed Heads Hospital he didn't look well at all. He was much thinner than he had been a few months beforehand, and he had a bandage around his head. George's dementia was in its advanced stages by then. Thus he kept excitedly showing us his drip needle in a childlike way, not understanding what it was and trying to pull it out.

On the way home we were all very upset and concerned about him. Though Grandad remarked about how George didn't look too bad, and that his own sprained wrist was much more of a concern.

A few weeks later (on Sunday July the 10th) we went down to the Gold Coast again to visit Brent's parents. George had left hospital by then and had returned to his nursing home, and our parents planned to quickly visit him before dinner that night.

Mum and Brent left me, Grandad and my younger siblings at Margaret's house with her, because a large number of visitors may have distressed George. Our parents also told us that they would bring in some food for us to eat afterward.

While we were at Margaret's house we were waiting for a longer time than we had initially been told. The house was quiet and tense, and it was very clear to us all that something was wrong. Then, Margaret got a phone call from Brent. It wasn't on speaker, but we mostly gathered that the situation wasn't at all good when Margaret kept asking urgently "Have you called the rest of the family and let them all know"?

Margaret put the phone down and told us that George had suddenly gone into organ failure and was having difficulty with breathing. As a result of that he had been taken into palliative care.

Yet once she had left to see George, Grandad said "It could be worse. Say, look at what damage my stroke did for me. I can't play the piano like I used to anymore". My siblings and I found those words to be extremely insensitive and inappropriate to say behind Margaret's back; and to say about George himself.

We ended up staying at Margaret's house overnight. Unfortunately we had no change of clothes to go to bed in. Though as it was rather cold, and in the middle of winter it didn't matter so much. I was not of course prepared and packed for staying overnight. Yet I did at least have my iPad and its charger in my bag. What's great about iPads is that they're a combination of virtually everything; notebook, computer, television, magazine, book, music player, alarm clock, and more.

Whenever I stayed down at Margaret and George's house I would sleep on the sofa in the living room.

At just after 4am Mum and Brent came back (Margaret was going to stay at the hospital) and said that George hadn't yet passed away, though he was very distressed. Despite having an advanced stage of dementia, he knew he was dying and knew that if he fell asleep he wouldn't be likely to wake up again.

They informed us that George was yelling out whenever he felt himself falling asleep and was very scared. But he had all of his family by his side, and his church minister came to visit him at 3am as well, for both comfort and to give his rite of passage.

He didn't end up passing away that night, and did fall asleep a few times over the following two days. We were informed by the nurses on the Sunday (when he was admitted into palliative care) that he would pass away any time from then to a few days afterward. Though George was determined to hang on for as long as he possibly could.

On Tuesday, July the 12th me, Mum, Kylie, Brent, Brendan, Dylan and Grandad were taken along to say goodbye to George. When we saw him in his bed that afternoon he did not look well. He was even thinner than he was while he was in hospital and the skin on his face was very tight. But the fear in his face was perhaps the most upsetting of all (a facial expression of which even I had noticed). He was looking up at the ceiling and his hands were trembling. In other words he looked absolutely petrified.

However when each and every family member spoke to him he looked at them with full attention. Every one of us said anything we could think of to comfort him. The nurses had tried putting on classical music but it seemed to make George even more distressed, because it wasn't an exercise that was familiar to him. Though when he got told that he would meet his late son again, along with his parents who he hadn't seen for many years, George closed his eyes (in a much more relaxed way) and calmly said "I know".

We visited Margaret and George's house once again that evening. I didn't bring along a bag large enough to hold my pyjamas. However I did pack (along with my iPad and its charger) a book to read and a

CHAPTER TWENTY-SEVEN

stress ball. This was because I was half expecting to end up staying down there for the night, and that ended up being the case.

Just like I did two nights beforehand, I slept on the sofa in the living room. It was so cold that sleeping in the sweater and jeans I wore during the day didn't matter much.

I didn't sleep too badly that night. However I was quick to wake up when our parents and Margaret arrived back from the nursing home just before 3am. The fact that Margaret had returned home told us that George had passed away.

Brent sat everyone down at the dining room table and told us that after they realised the classical music made him feel more distressed, they took the suggestion we gave about creating a more familiar environment instead. So when George's family were sat around him, they talked about things they usually spoke about, which were about riding motorbikes and watching MotoGP on television. This calmed George down immensely and after a short while he looked over at them, took a deep breath and then he decided to let go at last. There was a long stretch of silence and tears at the table.

At 4am it was time for us to return home. Margaret and George's house was an hourlong drive from our house, and Brent (like always) had to be at work early that day. Despite them being very cold, winter mornings are beautiful visually. We were going through a cold snap at that time, and while we were driving home there was misty fog and sparkling frost on the ground. This always looks so picturesque in the pink and gold colours of sunrise.

Sunsets never create this visual effect because we never have fog or frost on the ground at the end of a day. It's only ever at nighttime when it gets cold enough for us to experience those two things during winter.

On Thursday, July the 14th we had another challenging day. Yet it was challenging in a somewhat different way from two days before. We were due to take Grandad to the doctor that day to get his medication reviewed. Yet, first thing that morning we found him at the table fully dressed with his money pouch strapped around his waist.

He initially seemed quite fine. But then he unexpectedly brought up some personal issue with Jessica to provoke an argument. Though Jessica kept her cool and didn't say anything, because she knew exactly what Grandad was trying to do, and this wasn't the first time he had done something like this.

Yet Grandad persisted with his idea and then yelled about how he was fed up of being treated the way he was in our house, fed up with being ignored and that he was going to take himself to the doctor. As he was leaving he also gave a remark about how we must have loved and cared for (in his words) 'Saint George' more than him, due to us having to frequently include his name in conversations over those past few weeks. From there he slammed the front door shut and stomped out of the house and up the street.

At that time we were doubtful that he would be able to walk up to the doctors' surgery and cross the road in peak hour traffic. Though as mum was not his carer and he was a grown adult, she couldn't legally stop him from making the decision of taking himself to the doctor.

Yet mum called the receptionist out of concern (of whom she's well acquainted with) just as he stormed out of the house. She mentioned to her that he had vulnerabilities and asked if it would be okay for them to give her a call if he didn't arrive within an hour. Though 15 minutes later we were surprised to receive a phone call saying that he had arrived safe and well at the doctors' surgery.

It turned out that for several weeks Grandad had been secretly planning to leave, and had been looking online for places where he could live. His planned actions for the day had been to start an argument in the morning, storm out of the house, catch a bus to the place where he wanted to live, and put a deposit on a room there.

In the evening Grandad was driven to our house by a person of whom he was able to give our address to. Then (after knocking a happy tune) he said to us at the door "I don't want anything to do with you, as I don't have any family worth knowing, and living in your home surely isn't a bed of roses".

So Mum and Brent took him to the hospital, and they were told that he could stay there until it was time for him to move into his new house. The place he chose was at least an hour's drive from where all of his friends and family lived. His plan was to completely distance himself from everyone he knew.

Though he needed us to help him move his furniture and belongings from our house to his, and he deliberately chose the day of George's funeral to be as difficult as he possibly could. Once Mum and Brent had done that after paying our respects to George, we never heard any words from Grandad again.

George's funeral was on Monday, July the 18th, which was also one of his grandsons' birthday. Early in the morning we arrived at his local church and met up with other friends and family. This event was different from every other funeral I had previously attended, because it didn't involve an open coffin and it was a burial rather than a cremation.

This funeral was a very sad event and many tears were shed. A large number of people came up to the front to share their happiest memories of George. Towards the end of the service something very mysterious happened. Half of the many guests there (including myself) heard the hymn 'Amazing Grace' being played. As there wasn't an organist present at the time, we initially assumed that it was a digital recording. Though when people were expressing how beautiful it was to hear that hymn being played so expertly and appropriately, the other half of the guests were very confused because they didn't hear it being played. So for nearly half an hour we were passionately debating amongst each other about whether 'Amazing Grace' was played or not.

Though the debate concluded with the fact that 'Amazing Grace' was not played as no music was set up to be included, and a digital recording of the whole service revealed that there was no moment at all which included this hymn.

However Margaret and a couple of other family members expressed that 'Amazing Grace' was always George's favourite hymn, and that it was his strong desire to have it played at his funeral when the time came.

Whenever I listen to and/or read the words of 'Amazing Grace', I'm always interested as to whether George ever did become lost and then found his way by having faith in God. But after saying that, he did write an autobiography of his life many years beforehand, and he apparently got up to so much mischief in his childhood and teenage years. So all that can be asked and said here is "who knows?"!

After the service we made our way up to Southport Cemetery. George and Margaret had decided to be buried either side of their late son Kym, who was killed in a 1991 helicopter crash. We finally watched George's coffin being lowered down into his grave, and we then showered rose petals on top.

Then it was time for him to rest in peace, and to continue his existence through the next phase of his life journey. During the time when we are alive, this part of our existence is so mysterious and unknown that we can only ever call it 'the afterlife'.

Throughout the following couple of weeks I worked on adjusting myself to life without George and moving on after the sadness. As well, even though it was a very different kind of goodbye, I worked on getting over the hurt and anger of mum's father abruptly leaving us, with his final words of "I don't have any family worth knowing anyway".

Though in stark contrast, exactly two weeks after the funeral (Sunday, July the 31st) a very happy day occurred for me. Firstly, due to it being both *Harry Potter* and JK Rowling's birthday, the screenplay of *Harry Potter and the Cursed Child* was available to buy (as a book) in stores; and secondly, that was to be the evening when me and Markie's *60 Minutes* episode would air on Channel 9.

Unfortunately we had a very busy day with a few necessary errands to run. Therefore we couldn't make it to the store until 4pm, when they had (apparently) sold out of all copies of the book I wanted. After nearly an hour, I had been told by literally every bookstore and variety store in the mall that there were no copies left.

Even though I knew that they would restock very quickly (and I would therefore have a copy of *The Cursed Child* within a month regardless), I did still feel disappointed because I had been looking forward to reading that book on the day. However I then reminded myself that I had another exciting event to look forward to that night, which most people never get the privilege of experiencing. So I turned to leave the mall with feelings of acceptance, for the fact that me and everyone else in the world can't always have everything that we wish for.

Though just as I was doing that, incredibly, I saw Brent walking up to me with a copy of *The Cursed Child* in his hands!

What had happened was that a few staff members at Big W had taken a book aside hours beforehand to read themselves. While Brent was buying a new exercise bike for our home gym he asked the man serving him if there were any copies of *Harry Potter and the Cursed Child* left, as his daughter (myself) wanted to buy one.

Brent was then told that they did have one left, and that they'd give it to me. When he went to the main counter to buy the book, an employee who I spoke to earlier asked Brent if he'd been walking around for hours holding it. Yet when he told her that there was one in the back of the store, she laughed and said that she had no idea!

That same night, the additional event which was positive was that I got to finally see the *60 Minutes* episode featuring my story. As mentioned earlier, filming was done of me and Markie at the UCI, and was then followed by footage of me at Universal Studios and of Markie ice skating in her home state of Wisconsin. There was also footage taken of me at home with my Lego Village, as well as of me in the kitchen and dining room having a cup of tea. Once the story aired we were very happy with the way it had all come together.

By August 2016 I had already started doing public talks via YouTube and also at local seminars. As a result of that, several friends and family members had suggested that it would be a good idea for me to join Toastmasters. Toastmasters is very much like a course where we learn skills about public speaking of various kinds. We begin with a Competent Communicator course where we're taught a bit of everything in regards to being a speaker in general. Once we've finished those ten assessment speeches we then move on to the advanced manuals, where we can choose to learn more specific techniques. Now Pathways has been introduced. Though members who joined beforehand can continue working on the traditional manuals for a few more years.

I've now completed my Competent Communicator course, as well as the first of the three advanced courses, and have retained my title of ACB (Advanced Communicator Bronze). My intention is to continue doing Toastmasters, because there are always new techniques to learn with public speaking, and if it's not practiced regularly speaking skills do gradually become rusty.

A month after joining Toastmasters (on Friday, September the 2nd), I did a 90 minute talk at the University of Queensland. This involved me speaking to a class of students. The talk was for a friend Shane Scott, who's a course convenor in the field of Foundations of Social Work Practice in Disability. The talk ended up going very well, and many of the students told me afterwards that they expected a boring seminar, yet were amazed at how enjoyable it ended up being! I was very thankful for that!

Then, there was another talk I did (which was on Tuesday, October the 4th) where I was honoured with the privilege of being on an expert panel, in regards to autism and anxiety at a local seminar. My role was to speak as a person who literally lives with autism 24/7; and from there I was required to use the skills I had learned from Toastmasters (and previous public talks) to discuss what my challenges were articulately. I was very nervous when I was expected to do this for the first time. Yet afterward I was very pleased and thankful when I heard that it was received well by the audience.

Then, a month later was the 2016 US Presidential Election. For that I had to do a few surveys for the UCI, which were given throughout the whole month of November. These were all done via email. Firstly I had to predict how I would feel if Donald Trump or Hillary Clinton won the election. Then as soon as the election had happened, I had to give my feelings in regards to the actual outcome, and the researchers compared them to my hypothetical feelings given a few weeks beforehand. Finally I was sent another email weeks later which required me to cast my mind back to the election, and my responses were compared to how they were previously (which meant that all together I had to give my feelings for the future, feelings of the present moment and feelings about the past).

At the beginning of another busy month of 2016 (December) my previous Optus contract had ended. This was great news because I could then get a new iPad Pro and a pair of Bose headphones. I needed an iPad Pro for better video quality when it came to my Skype talks and interviews. Though I chose the one with an 11 inch screen so that I could still fit it into my handbag or backpack. As for the Bose headphones, I needed some that were soft to wear for long stretches of time, such as for when I was traveling (on long car trips or flights). Unfortunately AirPods and all other kinds of in-ear headphones don't work well for me, as my ears bleed and get infected every time I use them. So once I had left the Optus Store, I was holding both an iPad Pro and a pair of Bose headphones, which I was very excited about.

On Sunday, December the 4th we were out all morning and afternoon, but I managed to post a picture on social media of the purchases I got from the Optus Store the previous day. Optus themselves even commented on my Twitter post saying that enjoying my new iPad Pro was an absolute must. I responded by saying that I sure would enjoy it, and I also mentioned about how I always get my iPads from the two year contracts they offer. Optus then sent a lovely message thanking me for that.

When I came back home there was one more surprise in store for me. The *60 Minutes* episode featuring my story did so well in July/August that it was unexpectedly broadcasted for a second time that night! I was delighted to hear this news! At the end of 2016 (and after *60 Minutes*) I believed that there would be no more media events for me. Yet in a mere few months my story was set to unexpectedly go viral again, just like it had done in October, 2015.

CHAPTER TWENTY-EIGHT

DOING CONSTANT MEDIA INTERVIEWS IS A FULL TIME JOB

Sunday, December the 11th, 2016 was my 27th birthday, and just afterward (on December the 14th) I had my first MRI brain scan (at the University of Queensland). Normally my tests with them are done at the St. Lucia campus. Yet this MRI had to be done at the Herston campus, next to the Royal Brisbane and Women's Hospital. Just like I did with my previous MRI (at the University of California) I was required to lay as still as possible inside the machine for a stretch of time. However this time I had to do so for a slightly longer duration.

While I was inside the machine (still trying to keep as still as possible) I had to answer some memory related questions displayed on a screen above me. I couldn't wear metal inside the machine. But I was given goggles with lenses in them, so that I could read the screen properly. Scans were done of my brain every time I performed a memory puzzle. Most of the puzzles given to me were short-term memory related. Those kinds of memories are somewhat weaker than my long-term ones. For some very strange reason my memories become clearer as they get older.

Yet once I had completed the tests for that day, I was told that my short-term memory ability was actually a little bit above average! It just seemed poor next to my long term memory which was exceptionally strong. Though my photographic memory definitely isn't above average!

On Wednesday, March the 8th, 2017 (one day prior to Brendan's 18th birthday) I had a talk at the Cornubia Probus Club. That was another event which ended up going very well. There I spoke for nearly an hour about how I worked, and continued to work through my life challenges. My speech at this venue also got marked off as an assessment speech (from my Toastmasters Competent Communicator manual) by my club mentor, who attended the talk; and who was also the person of whom had suggested my name to the venue in the first place.

A month later (on Thursday, April the 13th) I gave a very similar speech at the Springwood Probus Club. I must add too that the meeting was held at a church building on Barbaralla Drive. Many years previously, I'd often mistake this exact same place as being our house, at the age of four. Prior to when we moved into our current home (when I was five years old), we lived in a townhouse off Barbaralla Drive. This caused me to experience an early childhood flashback, just as I had arrived there to do the speech.

It was an amazing experience for me to actually see what was inside that church building which I had mistaken as being my house. Though so many years had then passed that the furnishings were most probably very different.

In April of that year something else happened which was completely unexpected. OMNI/Vocal Media had recently started a public blogging platform where anyone could submit a 600–1000 word piece (in a variety of different subject areas). Once the blog receives admin approval the writer gets paid for the number of views the piece gets.

Anyhow, I received a Twitter message from Vocal Media during that April, in which they explained who they were and what they were about. At that time they were sending messages to people of whom they felt would be interested to start blogging on their site. They also asked us to help spread the word of this new platform, by encouraging as many people as possible to use it.

My first blog that I submitted to them was titled *I Can Remember Back to when I was a Newborn Child*. It was approved by the following morning and was posted on the site, so I could share the link on my social media. The places I shared the link on were Twitter, Facebook and LinkedIn. One of my Facebook friends (Nina) ran a very popular page and site called *Kidspot*. Nina really liked the blog that I had written, and she asked me if it would be okay for her to share it on her site.

My blog had been posted on Kidspot straight away, and I was

absolutely amazed by the amount of people who liked and shared it! My friends and cousins who had young children (and followed the Kidspot page) sent me posts and messages saying that it was amazing how they could find my name, story and photos in such random places! As my blog was shared so quickly, I didn't have enough time to tell everyone about it beforehand!

Two days after my blog had appeared on Kidspot, I noticed that I had gotten over a thousand new likes on my Facebook page *Superior Autobiographical Memory Australia*. That's when I approached my mother (who was the only person besides myself at home on that day) and said that something must have been going on somewhere.

My mother's the best person I know at finding media stories published about me on Google. So she got onto her iPad and discovered that *BabyCentre* had shared the blog of mine that Kidspot had posted. The surprises didn't stop there either. First thing next morning I received a message from *Daily Mail* asking if they too could share my blog that I had written. After replying to them with a message of yes, I was getting requests once again from media all over the world by that evening.

Just as it had been previously in 2015, this experience of a story of mine going viral was a sudden and enormous rush of work. However unlike 2015 I had gained more coping strategies over the course of nearly two years. So I was a little less overwhelmed than I was the first time.

From April the 24th, 2017 through to early 2018 I was kept very busy by doing many different kinds of media interviews. These included television, radio, newspaper, magazine and online stories. Throughout that particular time frame I did over a dozen individual interviews, both locally and internationally (thanks to modern technology and the availability of video calls via Skype). So it would be impossible to give all the details of each and every one. However, below are the highlights of those which didn't get lost in the editing process.

On Sunday, April the 30th I did my second talk on the *Sunrise* breakfast show. Just like I did a year and a half beforehand, it was a 3am start for me and my nerves were extreme.

Though when we arrived at the Channel 7 studio, my family and I

CHAPTER TWENTY-EIGHT

were entertained by a friendly stray chicken who (we were told) enjoyed checking in (or perhaps we should say 'pecking' in) to the goings on within the studio! The humour of all that lightened me considerably, and even though I was interviewed alone on the show this time, I was in a very calm state of mind throughout the segment.

After I did my interview we headed down to Dreamworld, to celebrate the success of that morning's experience. I'm so glad that Dreamworld is home to what is now Australia's largest Lego Store, and I bought myself the Lego Creator Christmas Train as a personal treat. Also, it kept coming back to me throughout the day that it was exactly one year since I had been filmed at the University of California for *60 Minutes*. Eastern Australia is a date ahead of the west coast of the US.

A few weeks later I did an interview for *Good Morning Washington* on Thursday, May the 18th. That interview was to be done via Skype, yet I was told that an earpiece was additionally required for the talk. As I didn't own an earpiece at the time, I needed to go out and buy one that day. It is true that devices which are inserted into my ear cause reactions after a short while. However this interview wouldn't require me to wear it for very long, and nothing else could be used.

But this was nowhere near as easy as I had expected it to be. All of our local electronic stores were unsure as to what would be required. Though from doing previous interviews at studios, I had gathered that a Bluetooth earpiece was what I needed.

Yet this information still wasn't much help to many of the local electronics store personnel we came across. In fact there was one store worker who had no idea what a Bluetooth device was and insisted that an external speaker was what we needed. As for Skype he only knew that it required a webcam. However he believed that it wouldn't work without both an external speaker and an external microphone. As well, he said that Skype could never be used internationally. After telling him that I had used Skype countless times before (during times when I did UCI talks), he told me to "shut up and stop talking sh**".

Mum, myself and the fellow store manager found that to be incredibly rude.

So while he was carrying on, I turned to my mother and said that we should go to someone who had a better understanding of technology, and someone who knew what they were talking about. Then we abruptly walked out of the store before he'd even stopped talking. Diplomacy didn't matter here, given that his own manners during that meeting were much worse than what I used with him. His fellow store manager even rolled his eyes, and gave us an approving nod.

After several hours of visiting countless stores, we reached a kiosk (which sold electronic devices in our local mall), and finally came across a person who knew and had exactly what we needed, which ended up being a bluetooth earpiece. It was indeed the correct device and my interview with *Good Morning Washington* (at 1am that night, Brisbane time) went really well. My family and I also liked how there was a medical expert on the show alongside myself; who assured the audience that HSAM is a true condition (despite its rarity), and that I had been diagnosed with it by a credible team of neurological experts with decades of experience.

Moving on to Sunday, June the 11th, 2017 I did an interview for another Australian breakfast show, *The Today Show*. This talk involved me and my family having to go to the Channel 9 Studio first thing in the morning. I was quite nervous before the interview and while I was sat at the desk ready to go on air, those nerves gathered considerably.

The talk generally went along very smoothly, and the only exception was at the very end. Just like I did on my first *Sunrise* talk, my mind went blank by nerves when I was asked to recite the first page of Chapter 14 of *Harry Potter and the Prisoner of Azkaban*. I even voiced that I had a blank while on air. Though *very luckily* I was able to recite the page just before the segment ended. Which was an absolute godsend for me, and I don't even want to imagine the consequences if that weren't the case!

Afterward we celebrated that time by visiting our local Build a Bear store where I made a rainbow coloured creature named Bonnie. Our intention was to recreate the happy celebration I had almost three months previously, when I spoke on *Sunrise*. Though fortunately, just as it was after I had done that *Sunrise* interview, it didn't take much effort to feel happy; from a combination of relief and positive satisfaction.

Once we arrived back home however, there was a slight downfall within me that I had to momentarily experience. My mother went online and discovered that an article titled 'I've had a blank' had been published by *Daily Mail*, in regards to the *Today Show* interview I had done earlier that day!

I initially felt like my stomach had clenched and turned into solid stone! Yet when my mother had read the entire article, they eventually mentioned that I got the words right in the end, and I literally thanked God that I did! This gave me much more relief. Though I did still feel a little bit embarrassed about my mistake throughout the rest of that day! But after a few days I completely got over it and my feelings returned to normal. My family, friends, therapists and HSAM researchers did also assure me not to worry about this, as reciting the *Harry Potter* books isn't a part of my HSAM anyway. As a child I (purposely) rote learned the words of the *Harry Potter* books to enable me to read myself to sleep with my eyes closed (as an aid for insomnia). Yet on (brief) live shows reciting those books is an interesting thing to quickly show and display; even though this technically involves semantic memory instead of autobiographical memory.

On Tuesday, June the 14th I had a BBC radio interview scheduled for that night (nighttime in my timezone and lunchtime in the UK). This was to be a cross studio broadcast from my local ABC station. However once we arrived there, we were told that the interview had to be rescheduled, due to there being rolling coverage of the Grenfell Tower fire. As this was breaking news, it was unexpected.

When we got home, we watched the news and footage of the tragic event and it was absolutely heartbreaking. House fires have always terrified me, and also my sister Jessica lives in an apartment. The dangers and benefits of living in an apartment and living in a house will of course be equivalent. Though my absolute worst fear whenever I'm in a high rise building (even a hotel suite that isn't on the ground floor where there's an easier escape route) is of a fire engulfing the building and trapping me in there. Underground carparks give me those uneasy feelings too, especially after I saw that news story as a seven year old, where there had been an explosion inside one of them on George Street.

Yet a couple of weeks later my BBC radio interview had been

rescheduled (with success) to occur on Tuesday, June the 28th. This story was aired at lunch time in the UK, which was very late at night in Brisbane.

Yet while I was in the green room, just prior to when I was talking for an hour in one of the Tardis rooms (which are used for cross-studio radio broadcasts at the local ABC studio), it was very relaxing to watch the lights and the city itself gradually fall asleep. It was a very pleasant interview as well, which put me in a comforting frame of mind for a solid few hours of sleep once I had returned home.

Due to living in a reasonably small city, there was no traffic on the roads late at night when we were returning home. Also, I must say that it always amuses me to see traffic lights giving their usual timed signals when there are no cars waiting by them. In fact, in various suburbs local to me, certain traffic lights are turned off during late night/very early morning hours for this reason (if it is safe to do so). Therefore, as a result of all that we made it home for 2:30am and went to bed straight away.

A month later I visited the same studio again for an episode of ABC Brisbane Evenings. There I did a long interview while playing a game of pool. As our minds were focused on the questions for the interview, neither me or the presenter managed to get very far with that particular game! However it was a really nice experience which ended with my song of choice. Just prior to leaving home that night I was asked for a song that reflects my life. The first that came to mind was 'Karma Chameleon' by The Culture Club. I was then asked why I chose that song. In truth I much prefer older songs than those beyond the year 2000, and my favourite decade for music (with lyrics and not classical) is the 1980s due to the intense passion contained in many of the songs.

Over the following couple of months, things were (reasonably) quiet for me. Then, in early September of 2017 I did a second talk for my friend Shane Scott's class at the University of Queensland. There I spoke for an hour and a half about my general life story in regards to all of my disabilities, which concluded with 30 minutes of questions and answers. It ended up going well, and those who were present for my talk a year beforehand said that they had really noticed how much Toastmasters had improved my speaking skills!

Later on in September of 2017, I visited the newly established *Store of Requirement* (a store that solely sells *Harry Potter* and *Fantastic Beasts* merchandise) in Brisbane for the first time. This store is located in the suburb of Samford which takes just under an hour to drive up to from my house. However the *Harry Potter* theme park in Hollywood is a 14 hour flight away. So I was absolutely thrilled about having a *Harry Potter* themed place much closer to home. The family who run the Store of Requirement are such wonderful people, and now they've also opened a store down in Melbourne.

The following month (October) was a very eventful month for me in 2017. Another one of my blogs, *Through the Eyes of a Toddler*, went viral worldwide. So for the first few weeks of that month I was kept very busy again with constant emails, social media messages and interview requests. It wasn't yet sweltering hot, though the Spring temperature was at a perfect level to sit outside in the garden with my iPad and a citronella candle in the evening. Thus I was relaxed and calm enough to answer each and every question I received on Twitter. Both myself and the people I was communicating with were very happy about my commitment and enthusiasm!

That month, I also participated in the International Speech contest for Toastmasters. My speech was titled 'Rising From the Ashes', and described my life journey from near hopelessness to developing a sense of direction in my life. The area competition was to be held on Saturday, October the 28th. A week prior to that day, I did a rehearsal at my home club.

After I gave the rehearsal speech one evening, another Toastmaster then took me into the kitchen area and told me that I would never be able to win a contest because I have a disability. Though he said that it would be good to learn from the experience of 'losing the contest', as all of the mistakes made would help me to correct my severely deficient communication skills.

Those certainly weren't the best words of comfort to give to a first time contestant of a Toastmasters competition, nor any other kind of competition. But I was still determined to give it a go, because if there is one thing I don't believe in, it would be to simply give up. To give up means to fail, and I was not at all willing to make that choice.

Even though I was mostly expecting to not achieve a place, I began the morning of the event in good spirits. The weather was beautiful and pleasantly balmy, and the area contest was held in a quaint town hall in the countryside. All of this put me into a very nice frame of mind. When the time came to do my speech I put in my best effort, despite knowing that it wasn't 100% perfect.

Once the time came to announce the winners, the third and second places were initially given. That's when I resigned myself with a feeling of happiness for giving it a go. Yet when first place was announced I was shocked to hear that I had won the contest! This put me through to the second round, due to be held in March of 2018.

Additionally, in November of 2017, another pleasant surprise came for our entire family. On Thursday, November the 17th I received an email from an independent film maker, Sari Braithwaite. Sari had read an article published by Trent Dalton in *The Australian* newspaper, which was about myself and my family members here at home. From reading that, Sari was very keen on creating a slice-of-life documentary film about how we all successfully live together, as a family of five adult children with disabilities (and with a father who has severe dyslexia).

At first, Mum stated that it would be a hoax, as none of us thought that a film company would ever be interested enough to make a movie about our lives. However once we had taken a risk by going forward with this request, we discovered that it wasn't a hoax after all; and our film *Because We Have Each Other* is due to be premiered at the Melbourne International Film Festival in August, 2022.

The following year of my life (2018) was set to be the busiest year that I've had to the present day. Hence the reason for why it is the largest chapter of this memoir that I've written.

CHAPTER TWENTY-NINE

ACCEPTING THAT I'M NOT QUITE READY FOR FULL INDEPENDENCE

Things went very well for me throughout the following few weeks, and when my 28th birthday came around I really enjoyed the day. It fell on a Monday in 2017 and Jessica came and stayed for the day, with a gift of a silver necklace with attachable character wands from *Harry Potter*. We had lunch at The Coffee Club, and then that evening my family gave me a jumbo sized *Harry Potter* plush, which was purchased at our local pop culture store, Zing.

Two weeks later was Christmas Day, and like almost every year it was a very good day for me. I was given a large pile of *Harry Potter* (3D) jigsaw puzzles as my gift. It was great fun for me to spend much of the day putting those all together. Yet the weather was steaming hot and very humid. Therefore while all of the roasts were being cooked for Christmas lunch, it seemed to add even more heat to the house! We have several fans but no air conditioning, as both my mother and I experience allergic reactions to the chemicals it releases. Luckily though, that day ended by us having a thunderstorm which cooled the temperature down greatly.

While we were watching the rain and lightning I received a vivid flashback of Christmas Day in 2005, when it was hot and humid all day long, but had eventually cooled down with an evening thunderstorm. In subtropical Brisbane, thunderstorms almost always cool down a hot and humid day/night. Though occasionally, they can just make conditions even more humid (while the heat remains). Yet thankfully, the latter I mentioned isn't usually the case.

The first few months of 2018 were rather busy, especially for the very beginning of a new year. On Saturday, February the 3rd I had an interview with *Great Big Story* on CNN. This was done from home in Brisbane, and my interviewer called me from the US. However a tech guy came to my house that morning to record the interview. The story was published a couple of months afterward and I was very pleased with the end result. March and April of 2018 included much activity in various other areas as well.

Sunday, March the 18th was our Division Contest for Toastmasters. This was of course a little more intense than the area competition. For that year it was held at Griffith University. But in complete honesty, I didn't turn up with the expectation or desire to win. Everyone joins Toastmasters for their own individual reason, and the purpose for me joining was to learn public speaking skills rather than to win competitions.

I wasn't at all surprised or disappointed when I didn't receive a place after giving my speech. Though I was told that despite not being much of a performance speaker, my style would be ideal for doing TED talks!

This came from an audience member who works with TED speakers. Her words made me happier than I ever would have felt from winning the competition, because it had been my dream for a very long time to be an international TED speaker!

TED and Toastmasters emphasise very different styles of speaking. Yet there weren't any other places local to me who taught public speaking skills, and it's (mainly) in Toastmasters *competitions* where the two styles differ the most. However a significant number of assessments in Toastmasters do teach us how to give informative talks, which differ vastly from performance speaking. Performance speaking requires more unnatural and dramatic actions.

In the aftermath of the Toastmasters competition I generally felt immensely happy, and almost a week later I had a travel training day with my therapist. We walked up to the bus stop at the end of my street and then boarded a ride to our local mall. There I did some shopping at Big W for some new nail polish, of which I use to help stop me from biting my nails whenever I feel stressed. Then before searching Translink for a bus to take me back home I had a chai latte at The Coffee Club. Chai Lattes (with zero coffee) do a great job with enabling me to ground my mind; particularly in a busy mall with lots of noise and other chaotic stimuli, which overwhelms my senses.

Coffee never works like that for me because I don't like the bitter taste of it, and the same goes for alcoholic drinks because I don't like the bitter taste of them either. To this day I have never experienced drunkenness, as I've struggled to swallow even one sip of an alcoholic beverage. Just like coffee, I can taste even the slightest amount of alcohol in a drink, or anything edible of which it's been added to.

Later that night something very unsettling and shocking happened in regards to my brother Brendan. After polishing his beloved car he told us in the evening that he wanted to visit some friends.

Then just after 9:30pm we received a phone call from Brendan in which his voice was very muffled, and he was saying that he'd been in a crash and his car was completely destroyed. Mum and Brent asked Brendan where he was, and then they went out to go and see him. Just as they were about to leave we heard sirens racing down our main road, and mum said that she sincerely hoped that they weren't for Brendan.

The next two hours were very tense for those of us at home. At around half past eleven we received a call from mum saying that Brendan's crash was caused by him street racing. He was going so fast that he had lost control around a bend, his car flipped airborne and rolled three times when it landed. She said that it was a miracle that he wasn't injured or killed and that he'd been taken to the Princess Alexandra hospital for a checkup. When mum and Brent sent us a picture of what remained of his car, it was plain and obvious that this crash had not been an accident.

Our whole family were shocked (as he loved that car so much) and very disappointed about his actions. Brent even told Brendan that he had a horrible flashback of the time when his brother Kym died in a helicopter crash, and about how he was so incredibly relieved that he didn't have to experience that all over again with his son.

That incident ended up with Brendan being fined with Careless Driving. He lost his licence for 3 months. Then Brendan was put on a provisional licence, and was warned that if he did anything like this again he would be criminally charged.

Thankfully Brendan has used that incident to share openly about how irresponsible and reckless it is to be a 'hoon'. He also put in a lot more thought to find the reason for why he had done what he did. Brendan came to the realisation that the daring sensation of fast driving helped alleviate his mind from depressive feelings. From that he's now working towards getting a racing license, so that he can do so legally and more safely on a racetrack.

Easter in 2018 fell on the first day of April. Jessica came around to visit us that day for our usual Easter breakfast of hot cross buns. Then in the afternoon we went to see the new *Peter Rabbit* film at our local cinema. The Beatrix Potter tales were the first fictional stories that I read as a very young child. However the new film of *Peter Rabbit* was different from how I expected it to be. I expected it to be good. Yet I didn't initially know that I would end up literally choking with laughter throughout the entire film!

When we returned home I spent the rest of the day finishing my Easter Town on *Disney Infinity*. After watching *Nightmare Before Christmas* I made a town in the game for each of the holidays we celebrate, including my own version of Halloween Town. My enjoyment of digital sandbox games started with *Disney Infinity*, and from there I began using other games in addition. Nowadays, I'm building all six of the world's Disney parks in the well known sandbox game, *Minecraft*. I use that activity to ground my mind, and *Disney Infinity* was the precursor for me in regards to this. So after coming home that Easter from the busy cinema, it was essential for me to wind myself down by building my Easter Town in *Disney Infinity*.

Yet a few days later, we had another exciting event to look forward to.

That year the Commonwealth Games (where countries from the British Commonwealth compete in athletic events every four years) were held on the Gold Coast. The opening ceremony was on Wednesday, April the 4th, and we were extremely lucky to have gotten tickets to see it live.

CHAPTER TWENTY-NINE

In order to receive tickets we had to put in an order online, and then we waited to hear the news of whether we could then purchase them. It was all a process of luck. So we put in an order for the opening and closing ceremonies. We were then delighted to find out that our whole family had been successful in our application for the opening ceremony (which was the most favourable)! This good news came shortly after Brent and Brendan's successful application to be voluntary workers for the 2018 Commonwealth Games. Their job was to offer water and refreshments to the competing cyclists.

Every person who attended the games for all events had to arrive via public transport. Ironically our house is walking distance (less than 1km) from a busy train track, yet our nearest train station (Altandi) is a 20 minute drive away! Altandi was on a direct route to our final destination at Nerang. We were hoping to park there but unfortunately it was full. So we had to park at another station and then take a connecting train back to Altandi, and then another down to Nerang. By car, a trip down to Nerang is a 40 minute drive for us. Yet by train it seemed to take roughly half that time.

Once we arrived at Nerang station it was very busy with both spectators for the opening ceremony, as well as a few of the performers and athletes. There were a heap of buses taking groups of people to the stadium, and luckily we didn't have to wait too long (that time) for a bus to take us there. As we approached the stadium, the grandstand where we would be sitting came into view and my mother was a little bit concerned about how high it was! However I rather liked the look of it as it reminded me of the Quidditch World Cup in *Harry Potter*.

Entering the stadium required us all to be x-rayed and searched just like we do so in an airport. Then, once we were in the vicinity we each had a classic Australian meat pie for dinner. Mum had to bring a salad from home, as just about all of the food available for purchase had gluten in it. Once we had finished dinner we made our way up to our seats, which were right at the top of the grandstand.

Even though we didn't have the best seats possible, the ceremony was absolutely amazing! The presentation was all about the culture of the Gold Coast both for European settlers and the First Nations of Australia (we live in the Yugambeh Country). We were all treated to a corroboree with a Smoke Ceremony, which is a kind of spiritual cleansing. It was an incredible experience! The sound of a didgeridoo being played by an expert was absolutely beautiful and the smoke ceremony released all of the stress out of my body.

Throughout the rest of the opening ceremony I felt completely calm, despite the fact that we had a brief rain spell at one point, and our seats didn't have a cover to shield us! We were all drenched from that shower and I sincerely hoped that my iPad and iPhone in my bag weren't damaged! Luckily they were both okay.

As always in the Commonwealth and Olympic games, all of the countries with competing athletes were called into the stadium in alphabetical order. Dignitaries including our former premier Peter Beattie, the current Queensland premier, the current Australian Prime Minister, HRH Prince Charles and a few other important public figures gave speeches. Migaloo, the giant inflatable whale also made an appearance in the ceremony that night. There were a few fireworks which I have a phobia of, yet luckily there weren't many during the ceremony and I had my earmuffs with me.

Making our way back home was by far the most challenging experience of that night. While all of the dignitaries were leaving, every person in the grandstands had to remain there for over half an hour. When we were finally allowed out we had to queue up and make our way (very slowly) to the buses. As we were waiting, there was a band playing loud metal music which made me sincerely believe that the organisers wanted the crowd to get so fired up, that riots worthy of publicity would occur. Incredibly (and perhaps to the organisers' disappointment) everyone was well behaved and kept themselves emotionally stable while seething with annoyance.

Once we had finally reached a bus, we were taken from the stadium to the Nerang train station. It was past 1am when our train arrived, and it was almost 2am when we reached our destination at Altandi. Then we had a 40 minute walk to the other side of (the suburb) Sunnybank, where our car was parked. This late night walk was safe as we were a party of six adults. As well, having a black belt in Taekwondo gave me a little extra confidence. But I sincerely didn't want to jinx myself by thinking or feeling that!

Though we ended up not running into anyone dodgy and it was actually a very peaceful walk for me. In the middle of the night there's very little noise from traffic, and the only sound (apart from ourselves) we did hear whilst walking was the occasional hoot of an owl or two. It's such a shame that there are people around who make nighttime walks so dangerous. Once we finally reached the car we drove back home, and by the time we got into bed it was past 3:30am. But I did fall asleep quickly, and I had many more positive events to look forward to.

A little later that month I attended my first **ICAN Network** Teen Mentoring Camp. Friday, April the 20th, 2018 was wet in Brisbane and prior to setting off to Redland Bay (where the camp was held that year) I was rather nervous. Yet having spoken a fair bit previously with the other mentoring staff (all of whom had autism like myself and were very friendly), I felt much less nervous than I would have been otherwise.

Just before I left home with mum that night I almost had a meltdown, but managed to pull myself together with a combination of a Valium tablet and mindfulness exercises. It was a very wet night and we stopped by a pie shop near the campsite so that I could have dinner beforehand. The pie was very nice indeed and the delicious taste of it soothed my nerves even further.

Once we had reached the campsite mum supported me by carrying my suitcase and bedding into my cabin. We were both amazed about how nice and fancy the cabins looked there. Each had proper beds, a bedside table, and a window with curtains. In fact the whole place was much more like a resort than a campsite. All of my fears which came from negative school camp memories, were then immediately removed from my mind. Excitement about what seemed like a fun weekend ahead replaced most of that fear. Yet I was still a little nervous about how well I would do as a mentor and adult figure for a group of young teens.

However I had previously spoken to the kids I was mentoring (as well as their parents) on the phone a few weeks beforehand, and we seemed to get along very well. So once I met the kids in person, we were familiar with each other, and things ran very smoothly from then!

Me and another young woman were adult mentors for the green group (the others being red, yellow and blue), which was formed by five autistic teenagers aged from 14 to 17 years old.

This mentoring camp was a great opportunity for autistic teenagers to connect with each other, and also for us autistic adult mentors to connect with each other simultaneously. Just prior to bedtime I was involved in a discussion about astrophysics, relativity and blackholes. I thoroughly enjoyed this because I don't have a chance to talk to people about those topics very often. Most people I interact with tell me that it's very boring, and annoyingly the topic of conversation changes.

After having a very stimulating night, combined with nerves about the upcoming camp, I was very concerned about whether or not I would be able to fall asleep. Yet I made the decision beforehand that I would take a Valium tablet prior to bedtime on the two nights, and would make sure that I had all of the streaming apps on my mobile devices. So after the Valium I took a few hours previously, and by watching *Coco* for a bit on my iPad, I managed to fall asleep very quickly.

First thing the next morning we did abseiling and archery. I was far too scared to volunteer myself to climb down a 5 metre wall in a harness. However I was more than willing to do the archery activity. I'd never used a bow and arrow before, it was rather windy and I wasn't that good. But it was such a calming exercise to focus my mind on the target, and engage my efforts on attempting to shoot the arrow towards the correct spot.

After archery we had lunch and all of the adult mentors (and some of the teenagers) had to give a short speech about a life experience which involved a message of "I can do this, regardless of what negative criticism I got". My own speech was about how I refused to believe that I'd never be able to leave the house or have a job, and how my journey towards achieving that (to my best possible ability) had been a slow but successful process. Listening to everyone else's speeches was a fabulous experience for me, because I was inspired from both their speaking skills and their own personal life journeys.

That afternoon we did canoeing which was much more of a challenge. Beforehand I thought that it would be a relaxing activity, and I brought the right shoes and clothing. Yet while we were out in the lake our canoe felt as if it were going to capsize at any moment, the water was somewhat deep, and despite having the right clothes on I was still wearing my glasses. All of a sudden I got this terrible fear that I was going to both fall in the water and (especially) lose my glasses in that large, deep lake! That caused me to have a meltdown way off shore and in front of everyone. Once I had been calmed down, the embarrassment settled in and that made me cry.

However I didn't end up being shamed for being one of the adult supervisors completely losing control of my emotions, which is what I feared most of all. On the contrary, what ended up happening is that the kids and fellow adult mentors opened up to me even more.

I had also discovered from one of the kids that the new Hogwarts Mystery app which I had been waiting weeks for was available in the App Store. So once I had returned to my cabin I downloaded it and created my profile.

Once we had our dinner, we got ourselves ready for 'Dress to Obsess' night. The ICAN Network created 'Dress To Obsess' as an opportunity for every person with autism to embrace their favourite topic by dressing in a costume of that theme. Then, as a group everyone (in any way that's possible) gives a short speech about what their costumes and interests are. It's perfectly true that not every autistic person is verbal and/or feels comfortable with speaking to a group of people. So just wearing a costume in the theme of their interest alone is enough for this activity.

After 'Dress to Obsess' it was time for a movie before bedtime which was the Disney film, *Ratatouille*. While the teens were either settled by watching the movie or going off to bed, the adult mentors stayed up a little later to talk about the activities organised for the next day; as well as to purely and simply socialise with each other. When I finally went to bed on the last night of that camp, I felt quite sad that it had come to an end.

This was nothing at all like the difficult camps I had at school. In fact, I felt the same level of enjoyment with this as I did with my holidays overseas. I made up my mind quickly that I would do this mentoring camp all over again in a heartbeat.

Next morning everyone had to pack up their bags and belongings, then put them all into the hall. As well, the mentors had to check each and every cabin for anything that had been left behind. Once everything had been done and organised, it was time for one last activity before we went back home after lunch.

For our group it was Jacobs Ladder and I'd have to say that this was perhaps my favourite activity, if I had to pick a favourite. I wasn't the person climbing but I found that I really enjoyed working the ropes to pull our climber up the rungs. It wasn't a case of merely pulling the ropes. It was in fact a mathematical sequence which I had to do over and over, and I have a great interest in doing activities like that. Our team even ending up winning the game! That put me in a positive frame of mind once the camp was over. But even so, I wasn't expecting to be just as happy when things returned back to normal again.

However, a few days later, I received a pleasant surprise which restored my happiness after the 'end of camp blues'. In Australia we celebrate ANZAC Day on April the 25th every year. That date is a public holiday where we honour the work of current and past war veterans. This is done by us attending morning marches, and/or making or purchasing wreaths to place at memorials.

The largest ANZAC ceremony is held in Gallipoli, Turkey. That was one of the places where a great number of ANZACs (Australian and New Zealand Army Corps) tragically died in the First World War. The two historic battles from that war, which I learned (the most) about at school were those of Gallipoli and the Somme; even though there were many more battles fought in that single war and beyond.

However there are other marches held on April the 25th all over Australia/New Zealand, and that year (2018) we attended our local march. Eighteen years had passed since I last saw a veteran from the First World War, and now veterans from the Korean and Vietnam wars are the ones who are typically the oldest.

On ANZAC Day of 2018 the crew who were beginning to do filming and work for our family movie spent the day with us. After the march we had a fancy lunch at our house. During lunch I received a very positive surprise on social media, that I wasn't at all expecting.

CHAPTER TWENTY-NINE

After spending all morning at the march, I got a chance to check my Facebook messages when I got home. One new message appeared in my box and I opened it to check what it was.

Immediately I recognised the name Rahni Sadler, having previously watched the news for so many years. When I opened her message it was very pleasant, and additionally Rahni gave me some very exciting news!

She worked with a well known television personality, Andrew Denton. Rahni told me that he had been following my story since the very beginning of my media journey and that he was a huge 'fan'!

I was then asked to give her a call back whenever I was available. My parents were very excited too, as were the film production crew who were already with us that day for their own project. They expressed how wonderful it was that I would be doing an interview with Andrew Denton, and how they themselves had spoken to him before and that he was a lovely person.

When I called Rhani immediately afterwards, we were told that they'd love to have both me and my mother down in Sydney for an interview, a week from then. After we both enthusiastically agreed to this we were sent information and tickets for our flight, as well as our accommodation.

On the morning of April the 30th (exactly two years after being filmed at the UCI and exactly one year after appearing on *Sunrise*) I was a little bit nervous about the upcoming evening. Never before had I done a flight and then a television interview in the one day. It is a very scary experience to do for the first time.

That morning I had a psychology appointment, which was lucky for me, because I came very close to having a meltdown in the office. When my voice became louder than usual and I had speech which was more grammatically broken, my therapist gave me a grounding exercise to do which was very helpful. In fact, I continue to use this at other times when I am feeling the same way.

This exercise is called 'Leaves on a Stream', and it involves one imagining that they are sitting beside a flowing stream, then to visualise random thoughts coming into the mind (regardless of what they are) as leaves to simply throw into the water without further analysis.

Whenever I begin to do this exercise, I initially find that I'm throwing one or two 'leaves' into the imagined stream every second. Though eventually the frequency becomes less and less, and after a few minutes I feel much calmer.

Just after 1pm that afternoon, a car came to take us to the airport. By that time I was fully ready and calm, due to both my therapy session and having had a Valium tablet. Once we arrived at the airport it was easy for us to check in, as our flight tickets were sent to us on our mobile devices. Also, as it was a short trip we didn't have much luggage with us. So it was much like the weekend camp I had been on earlier that month. While we were waiting for our flight mum thoroughly enjoyed being in the business class lounge where we got to have a buffet lunch/dinner.

Our flight down to Sydney was an hour and a half, and then after arriving in our hotel room we spent a little bit of time there before going to the Channel 7 studio.

During the car ride to the studio, I was quite nervous again and was very quiet as I was going over my mental notes, in preparation for what I may have been asked on the show.

However as soon as we were greeted into the studio and shown our green room (where we had such nice company), all my nerves had vanished. Andrew Denton even came down to visit before the interview to greet us, make us feel comfortable and to go over what we would be asked on stage. After I calmed down, it was then my mother's turn to be nervous! She had no idea that she too would be on stage!

Yet mum was told that the way she was dressed was excellent. She was also given all the information she needed for what she was to say in the interview, and we warmly reassured her that everything was going to be fine.

When the time came for us to be on stage for the interview, both of us felt very calm and relaxed. Andrew Denton was so lovely to us, and he is a very intelligent and entertaining interviewer.

The session began with audience members asking me to recite pieces from the *Harry Potter* books, which ended up going very smoothly. Then me and my mother were asked questions about how our lives were with HSAM, autism and our typical daily living. An advantage of being one of two (or more) interviewees is that each can have short breaks, while the other is answering a question.

Both the show and the audience were truly delightful. After we had finished the interview I received yet another surprise! I was handed a Wrebbit *Harry Potter* jigsaw puzzle, which had only just came out; and less than a week before then I had wished to buy it at QBD (my local bookstore)!

After giving many thanks, I was asked one last question on stage. This was about whether it really was true that I could re-taste black forest gâteau (my absolute favourite dessert), whenever it was on my mind. In a previous interview, I had mentioned this very peculiar fact. Andrew then said that he liked my taste in food very much, and he presented me with a whole Black Forest gâteau in a box, for me to eat and share!

We woke early the following morning to take a beautiful walk through the Sydney Botanical Gardens, and then to the harbour where we boarded a ferry to visit Taronga Zoo. This trip was strongly recommended to us the previous night and it definitely was a really good experience. Despite having had a panic attack in the cable car due to it's small size and tight locks, my visit to the zoo was one of the happiest experiences of my life.

To begin with, we visited the reptile exhibit which (literally) had every kind of reptile and amphibian I could think of; and having grown up in Queensland I have heard of a vast number! Snakes are such beautiful creatures even though my mother is terrified of them, and I really enjoyed seeing many lizards and turtles that were different breeds from those we had at home as pets.

After we had finally seen and taken pictures of all the reptiles, we stopped at a cafe to buy an ice cream, and then while I was eating it we spotted two giraffes who were innocently looking over the wall at the sight of Sydney harbour. This was unlike many of us humans who take the beautiful view for granted, and look at the harbour mostly as a means of transport. As I was finishing my ice cream we saw a family of gorillas who were eating bananas. The mother was peeling her bananas and handing them to her young, while the father was sat all by himself surrounded by peelings and shovelling down all of the bananas he had.

At half past two in the afternoon we left the zoo to make our way down to the hotel, in order to check out and collect our bags prior to flying back home. Our return flight was much smoother than the one we had the previous night, and in just over an hour we landed in Brisbane.

Brent collected us from the airport, where I was delighted to see a small Lego village on display (of a QANTAS plane with its crew on a tarmac). During the drive home we told Brent everything that had happened, of which we hadn't yet mentioned on social media. This was due to confidentiality because the episode hadn't yet been released.

A month later, on Saturday, June the 9th, I received the news that my story on *Interview* (which was the name of the show I had just appeared on) would be airing at the end of the following week! This I shared with my friends and family immediately, and I was also then able to share the news publicly to advertise.

The episode of Interview on which I appeared first aired on Friday, June the 15th 2018. It ended up being a huge success. My friends and family enjoyed it, and it was fantastic to see that almost 90% of the social media comments were positive! By then I had gotten used to the possibility of negative and hurtful comments. But my friends still encouraged me to read the comments of this particular story, because most of them weren't only nice, but absolutely lovely.

The next day was Kylie's 21st birthday party (her actual birthday was on Wednesday, June the 13th). Even though Kylie was in her twenties, we had her party at Build a Bear because that's what she and the rest of her family/friends truly wanted.

Unfortunately, the usual Build a Bear which we visited had a party booked for that Saturday. Yet at the time there was also a Build a Bear kiosk at the Logan Hyperdome that was available. That shopping centre is roughly the same distance away from our home as Carindale. So it wasn't any more difficult for us to have the party there instead.

As well, there was enough space for Kylie's many adult friends/family (who also had various kinds of disabilities) to sit around, make a bear and enjoy the fun. I myself made a cream coloured bear named Faith.

For lunch that day we went to Sizzler, which was for the first time in nine years. Many of those restaurants had by then closed down, and Sizzler at the Hyperdome was the only one local to us that was still open. Yet I must say that despite the food not tasting that bad, I did get a little bored with eating the same things repeatedly. In our years growing up as a family there were *many* birthday celebrations we had at Sizzler each and every year.

Once we had celebrated Kylie's 18th birthday, I received some further exciting news! After seeing my story on Interview, the Maitland City Council contacted me with a request to speak at their upcoming breakfast event (for education in schools), which would be on the first of August. This was set to be my first interstate speech so I was very excited, as well as a bit nervous. But I was very keen to say yes to this event! Mum was very kindly invited along to support me as well.

Considering the fact that all five of mum's children have lifelong disabilities, she definitely has had a lot of constant work to do. Yet something came along very recently that has taken much of this immense stress and workload off her.

It was in the middle of 2018 when the NDIS (National Disability Insurance Scheme) rolled out in Queensland. The NDIA (National Disability Insurance Agency) is an organisation which gives eligible people with disabilities an annual block of (cloud) funding provided by the government. Only therapists and support services registered with NDIS can withdraw money from a person's funding. The purpose of NDIS is to accommodate the high expenses of therapy and all kinds of medical supports, in relation to an individual's disability. Yet for all of those things which every person is expected to pay for (such as transport, education, rent and general living expenses), they are understandably not covered by NDIS.

With my disability I require a lot of psychotherapy which was costing me a few hundred dollars a month (for each individual session), in addition to being on a lot of expensive daily medications. There were also other therapies I required but couldn't previously afford. So due to there being many expenses in my daily life, of which a person doesn't generally have to pay for, I was granted an NDIS package.

Though in the year leading up to my interview with the NDIA we did have a few worries and concerns. There had been much news about the arrival of the NDIS for a couple of years prior to it rolling out; and there had been a lot of talk about how the process was being slowed down by an inundation of people with autism applying for funding. As I myself have autism (which is my primary disability) we were slightly concerned that I would get rejected and knocked off the list as a result.

Yet when my NDIA interview eventually came up we presented them with all of the reports, diagnoses by psychologists, a letter from the therapist (who I was seeing at the time) in regards to my psychological state, and all the information of my goals and projects for the career I was developing.

My career goal at that time (as well as in the present day) did involve writing and public speaking. However I also had a very strong desire to create an organisation for teenagers and adults with autism (as well as other disabilities) where a self discovery program could be undertaken to enable each of our individual clients to find out where their true passion is. Then from there, educational and therapeutic sessions would be provided to each individual client so that they could discover exactly how they would like to use their passion in their life. This would be completely at our clients' own individual pace.

After receiving all of my medical information (which consisted of approximately fifty pieces of paper), they were very pleased. The whole purpose of NDIS is to provide funding for people with disabilities to work on becoming as independent as they can possibly be. Each plan lasts 12 months (occasionally 24 months) until another review gets done. In the reviews they go over how much of the previous funding was spent, and how much the person had been helped by the year's therapy and support services. Then it's determined how much funding will be needed for the next year, and as the person gains more independence and capability, less funding is given to them. Also, the funded money given to us can only possibly be used for its intended purpose, as our coordinator is in charge of all withdrawals.

We were very pleased to discover that the NDIA meeting was successful, and my initial year of funding was issued on Wednesday,

July the 4th. I must also say that I was very fortunate to receive an NDIS package. There are so many people I know with autism and other life-affecting disabilities, who have been incorrectly assessed by NDIA as not being dependant enough to receive funding by them. For instance, Brent has dyslexia to a level where he has a lot of difficulty with filling out medical and legal forms/documents. As well, dyslexia also affects a person's verbal speech, certain kinds of memory and ability to organise information. Yet the government doesn't give him any support whatsoever from NDIS, nor even the Disability Support Pension. So I do (and should) count myself as very lucky.

As we moved further into July, I began to feel nervous about a project other than the NDIA review. This was when my talk down in Maitland was coming much closer. Doing a paid speech for the first time is very scary. I had never even considered that fact before. It appears to be one of those things that only occur to us when we actually have to *experience* the situation, and to not merely dream about it happening.

That July, my deep inner feeling of insecurity even disguised itself as a completely different fear. In the final week of the month I had a restless night's sleep and woke in the early hours of the morning in a blind panic.

A fear suddenly entered my mind. This fear was that I was going to die in a plane crash, and that the tortuous story I was told as a seven year old was true. It was so intense that I was even shaking in my bed, and was scared that I'd have to make the decision of canceling my attendance at the breakfast, as well as canceling my trip to the US later that year. Having to do that would be extremely embarrassing, and it would make me feel and look like an absolute wimp.

Thus, my fear of the embarrassment of having to voice and act upon that decision, was just as intense as my sudden fear of being in a plane crash. So I reminded myself over and over that I had already flown a fair few times before, nothing had gone wrong, and the excitement of what was at the other end made all of those flights a happy experience. But in answer to this reassurance, my mind then told me "maybe this time you won't be so lucky". My anxiety also reminded me of the time when I stated that 'oo-na-nas' weren't real. Though after seeing that red hallucination in my room as a five year old, I was told by the sadistic person who created my fears of these monsters "You see I was right, oo-na-nas are real, you need to listen to me when I tell you that". This was the exact same person from my childhood, who lied to me about being the sole survivor of a gruesome plane crash. So my panicked and irrational mind was thinking "if he was correct about oo-na-nas existing, perhaps he was also correct about those horrific plane crashes".

As the 31st of July crept nearer those unsettling feelings escalated, to the point where I had no choice but to voice them. I even broke down in tears while I discussed those fears to my mother the night before our flight. Embarrassment made me feel even worse. Yet mum's advice soothed my emotions, in the exact same way as drinking a hot chocolate on cold winter's night does. Her words of "Becky, it will be fine, trust me" made all of those fears vanish.

When bedtime came I finally realised that my actual fear (disguised behind that all) was the speech. With that realisation I reminded myself that I had done plenty of speeches before, and that they were nothing to be afraid of. I fell asleep smiling, amused and laughing to myself. This time the words at the back of my mind were "all that drama just for a small issue like that"!

It was an early start the following morning, as our flight was just before 10am. So we arrived at the airport at quarter past seven to have breakfast beforehand. I myself had a blueberry muffin and a glass of orange juice. Muffins are very filling so I didn't need any more than one. Another thought that kept going through my mind was that it had then been exactly two years since the airing of me and Markie's *60 Minutes* episode.

Also, there was a moment after I had just finished my breakfast when a couple came over to the table next to me, and they had a baby. The baby then started crying. Brent was sat next to me while Mum was still waiting in line to buy her gluten-free breakfast. As I was hearing the high pitched wailing I turned to Brent and said "You know, if I couldn't remember back to when I was a baby myself, I wouldn't understand and tolerate their constant crying. I'd just find babies annoying".

Then Brent said "When you're a parent and live with them it *can* get really annoying at times". However after I replied with "I'd imagine it would be", I did acknowledge that living with my loud voice and my occasional meltdowns would also be extremely annoying. Brent laughed alongside me about this, and my anxiety about my trip in a small vehicle lessened even more with this lighthearted conversation we were having.

Checking in was very easy because we were only staying in Maitland overnight before returning home. Our onboard suitcases were all that we needed for this trip. It takes a mere 58 minutes to fly from Brisbane to Newcastle, and after all that panicking over the previous week, it ended up being the most beautiful flight I have ever had to date. In complete honesty there wasn't even a single moment of bumpiness. If my eyes were closed I wouldn't have even guessed that we were travelling in a vehicle, such as a car or an aeroplane.

I had purchased the new *Peter Rabbit* film to watch on my iPad while I was on the way down to Newcastle. However I found myself constantly looking at the picturesque scenery outside of the window. There wasn't a cloud in sight and all the colours of nature were in full view. But sadly due to the extreme drought most of the colours I saw were brown, orange and yellow, with barely any green and blue.

When we arrived at Newcastle airport, the weather was nice also. Our road trip (just afterwards) towards Maitland was mostly across the beautiful countryside. In my personal opinion the countryside is so much more picturesque than the busy cities are. This road trip took just over half an hour and once we arrived at our destination we felt very content.

We began our day there by checking into our hotel room which was very large and nice. About an hour later (after doing some mindfulness colouring to ground my mind) we left to go for a walk. The scenery truly was very beautiful.

The shops we went to look at were in and around The Levee. First I visited Preah Ko to buy some crystals (as gifts for my sisters and Dylan), along with some stress balls for myself. Then we visited Tomcat books and comics before having Subway for lunch. Luckily Mum was even able to get something that was gluten free.

After lunch we did some more exploring and shopping. One of the places we went to in the evening was the local museum and art gallery. Both mum and I love to look at historical exhibits and work by artists. Mum is currently writing books about the history (and especially the untold history) of Australia, so she thoroughly enjoyed looking at the museum. The artwork by local artists was absolutely amazing.

Eventually it was time for dinner. We used to have an Outback Jack's restaurant in our local area, but it closed a few years ago. Yet we were pleased that Maitland still had one open. We certainly weren't the only people to have dinner there that night, it was very busy indeed.

Both mum and I ordered a meal, and each ended up being so large that neither of us could finish our plate of food! Yet we enjoyed every bite we could eat, and took away our leftovers to have for breakfast the following morning.

The next day I got up early and did as much preparation as possible for my speech. When I first began doing talks I would write up a script, and then I'd work on memorising it all (I discovered that one hour is roughly 10,000 words). However once I started doing Toastmasters I learned a much easier way.

Reciting 10,000 words in a week is only possible if I put an extremely large amount of effort into the task, and if I have nothing else to do that week. But having to rote learn (by semantic memory and not autobiographical memory) all of those words in a short space of time does take so much energy; and also constantly having to work on memorising a long script only reminds me of how difficult the task is. That just makes the whole event even more stressful for me.

Those are the moments when I sincerely wish that I had been blessed with a photographic memory, where I could simply take a picture of a ten page document (in size 12 font) with my mind. It *is* possible for me to rote learn that amount of words in a (reasonably) small amount of time. However, given that my Short Term Memory isn't quite as strong as my Long Term Memory, I would need to give myself at least ten days for that task.

Yet at Toastmasters we're trained to give and construct every speech via mental notes, and preferably not by reading them from paper, or by using too many slides during a presentation. Rather than memorising a whole script, we prepare our speech by breaking it down into chronological sections.

So when we are writing up our presentation it's merely 3–6 sentences, each being our topics of discussion at certain times during the speech. A five minute presentation usually contains three sections and a ninety minute presentation will usually contain six sections. Also, in preparation we set ourselves a certain amount of speaking time for each section. For longer presentations we set ourselves more speaking time for each topic of discussion than we do with shorter ones. After doing various assessment speeches at Toastmasters, we're trained in such a way that we can always give a rough estimation of how many minutes we have been speaking on stage, without needing a clock or a watch.

My speech at the educational breakfast in Maitland was held in the town hall that morning. I was quite nervous when I walked into the venue. Yet after meeting the mayor, councillors, teachers, fellow speakers and school students before the event I felt much calmer. They were all such lovely people and children. Prior to the event, breakfast was served and I had a relaxing cup of English Breakfast Tea. Both hot chocolate and tea have such a calming effect on me. As mentioned before, coffee and alcohol never affect me that way. Before it was my turn to give a presentation, I enjoyed listening to the mayor's speech along with the young woman who was on stage just before I was. Once it was my turn to do a presentation I gave a combination of all that I had previously rehearsed, things which related to my struggle to fit in as a child (which was also covered in the speech prior to mine), and answers to questions the audience had given me.

As is always the case, when I began giving the speech to the audience, I felt my nerves slip away quickly and I was relieved that I didn't lose my thread. Once I had finished I had a happy 'buzz' inside me about having completed the presentation without running away in tears.

With all of those feelings I experience though, I am never fully sure about whether the audience liked my presentation until I get feedback. So I feel happy whilst I'm on stage at the end of my presentation.

Though when I return to my seat and sit down for a few minutes, I begin to feel a little nervous again.

However once the event came to a close, audience members were coming up to me saying that they enjoyed my presentation, which made me very pleased. A few even told me that they would love for me to talk at events of their own, and some even asked if they could have a photo taken with me.

By the time the event had completely finished it was nearly 12pm, so we decided that we should have an early lunch before doing some more last minute exploring and sightseeing. For that, went to the cafe at the museum to eat, and while we were there I received a very delightful message on social media.

The previous afternoon, I had posted some pictures on Twitter of myself by the Hunter river, doing shopping at the mall. It didn't take long for *The Maitland Mercury* to notice (within less than an hour) and contact me with a request for an interview! Both mum and I were amazed and happy!

My flight back home to Brisbane wasn't until past 6pm, and the airport was only small. So I was very happy to say that it was possible for me to talk with them, any time they were open on August the 1st. The journalists at the office were lovely to talk with and I had a fantastic time doing the interview.

All too soon it was time for us to travel to the airport and return home. It had been a while since I'd had a takeaway meal, so I decided to have Red Rooster for dinner. Mum of course also bought her dinner from there, as their hot chips were gluten free (without the chicken salt). Our flight departed just after 6pm and it was another smooth ride. On the 58 minute journey I watched *Peter Rabbit*, and I was very pleased that I seemed to have managed the experience without a meltdown, or any (noticeable) sign of anxiety.

However events changed somewhat at the other end, which made me feel very down about myself. Once we had landed in Brisbane I didn't have a meltdown, but I had something which is called a shutdown. What happened was that anxiety had crept up on me unnoticed during the past two days, and my anxiety doesn't disappear as time passes.

It almost always builds up until I have an explosive meltdown.

There was a reason why I wrote 'almost always' in the previous sentence. If I don't control every moment of anxiety with grounding exercises, I usually end up having a meltdown. But on this occasion I noticed my first ever shutdown.

After landing from this flight, I was so overwhelmed that I completely lost all sense of awareness and functioning. I wasn't saying or yelling a word. However I wasn't doing anything else either. I was completely unaware that twenty minutes had passed since we were able to disembark, and I was just sat motionless and thoughtless in my seat.

The moment when I became somewhat aware of my surroundings was when my mother was helping me stand up to get out of my seat. As I was being guided through the gate and airport, I began to experience anxiety from confusion. Finally when we were outside I was able to take myself away and sit by a wall.

In a near meltdown I asked my mother about what had just happened, as I was extremely confused. Mum then explained to me that I had been sat in my seat so long that the flight crew and airport staff had become suspicious and were forcing us to leave. Once I had processed all of those words I felt ashamed, embarrassed and scared. I had no idea how to control all of those emotions that had just washed over me.

As a result of that I ended up having a meltdown in plain sight of everyone walking in and out of the airport. That added even more feelings of embarrassment. For the rest of that night (as well as the following week), I struggled to accept the fact that despite being a grown adult I was unable to travel anywhere without a support person; especially interstate and overseas.

Though soon afterward there were other projects to focus my thoughts on instead, and they successfully distracted my mind from all of those negative feelings.

Almost a month after that, our family received some very surprising, extremely bizarre and even disturbing news. I was on Facebook one night updating my pages and a friend sent me a message asking about how Grandad was, as he hadn't heard from him lately. This was the grandfather who stormed out of our house two years beforehand, saying that he'd never speak to us again.

I then explained this situation to our friend and he was very sympathetic. He also let me know that he was concerned that Grandad had died, as he was failing to return all of his messages. The next day mum called the retirement home he was staying at, asking about his whereabouts and whether he was okay.

That's when the story began to unravel. Over the course of that day we discovered that Grandad had passed away nearly a month before, and it had been a fortnight since his cremation.

Though he insisted that he didn't want to let anyone know that he had died because he said that he had no family or friends worthy of paying respects to him. We also discovered that he had been saying horrible, slanderous things about my parents, which included claims that they had abused him while he was staying with us.

But we certainly weren't his only relatives of whom he hated with a passion. He truly felt after all that he had no family worth knowing.

When it came to attending medical appointments and taking his medications, he would never accept them. This was because he always insisted that he knew his own body better than any doctor did.

Yet a time came when he realised that he did indeed have heart failure. It turned out that the doctors were correct all the way along. Then as a result of him refusing earlier treatment, his cardiac issues had reached the stage of being terminal.

From discovering this, he had a desire to gain revenge on everybody he detested. The idea was that he wasn't going to have a funeral. Nor was he going to let any of his friends and family know that he died. The only people who seemed to know were the two owners of the retirement home, the hospital and the funeral home.

So, he had literally gone straight from the morgue to the crematorium, which was sad for us to discover despite how horrible he was to us.

We were also the ones who let his family in the UK know about his passing. All of them were feeling the same as we were. Why on earth would someone plan to end their own life like this as a way of spiteful revenge? They agreed with us that it was extremely weird.

Mum also felt it right to call her mother to let her know that Grandad had died. She had found her number in the telephone directory, and this would be the first time mum had spoken to Nana in two decades. It was a very uncomfortable but necessary moment.

Though Nana initially appeared to be pleased that mum had called her, but told her that there would be difficulties with passing along the information to Mum's sister. That was because neither Nana or ourselves had been in contact with her for several years, and it was unknown to any of us where she lived. Nor did any one of us know her phone number. This is still the case to this day.

On Sunday, September the 23rd we went out to Clifton to visit Nana. Clifton is a two and a half hour drive from our home; out past Warwick and close to the city of Toowoomba. On the way much of the scenery looked like vast expanses of empty and relatively flat land. I quite enjoyed the road trip though, as over the course of my lifetime I had gotten rather bored of constantly seeing modern, built up and heavily populated cities.

I hadn't seen Nana in twenty years, and she hadn't seen me since I was a child. Yet I had an enjoyable time visiting her that day. I even spotted the same chair I was sat in at the age of three when I hurt my leg, and that photo has been published in a large number of my media stories. So we took a new photo of me sitting in that very chair as an adult…

Then before we knew it, we rolled into October of 2018, and it was the busiest month of the year for me. That's saying a lot given that 2018 was perhaps the busiest year of my life so far. By saying that I was 'busy', I'm emphasising how I was doing various things which were more unexpected, and not usually a part of the life I've become accustomed to living.

That month I had four exciting events which were two local speeches, a radio interview and a family holiday (which extended into the first few weeks of November).

Being busy almost always brings excitement, stress and fun into my life. I don't like to escape my comfort zone, however I do love to challenge myself (especially with work, study and personal growth). This is the main reason for the unexpected answers I give people when they ask me questions about whether I ever feel overworked, or even bored. As a side note I've got to say that I never really experience boredom. Even if things do become mundane for a few seconds, it doesn't take long for my mind to turn it around into something that I find entertaining.

The radio interview I did was for Triple M in Melbourne, and was done via a cross studio broadcast in Brisbane. This happened on Wednesday, October the 17th and was yet another enjoyable experience. To date, I've found that every interview I have done has included something new for me to learn.

Within this interview I had a new experience of answering on-air questions from the audience. Prior to doing this I was asked if I was okay with doing that. Though I almost immediately said yes, because I had then reached a stage where I was generally unaffected by reading public comments (both positive and negative) on social media posts of my stories.

Though, I must admit there were still *some* nerves within me. However I was lucky to have been asked such wonderful questions from the audience, and not one of them was negative. At the end of the segment I expressed how happy and thankful I was about this!

As mentioned above, I also had two speeches in October of 2018, prior to our family holiday.

The first speech I did was for an **Autism Mates** event that was held on Saturday, October the 21st. Autism Mates is a non profit organisation which was created by a parent Randa Habelrih and her son Richard, who is autistic like myself. As an organisation they provide events that enable autistic children and adults to express themselves, and connect with likeminded people. They also hold charitable events to assist us with contributing our talents and skills to the world.

Autism Mates is based down in Sydney, yet Randa and Richard travel to take their fantastic work to multiple parts of Australia and across the world. In October of 2018 they came up to Brisbane, and held an event for autistic speakers (including myself) to give a talk about how autism influences their life, in a positive way. All of the teenagers and young adults gave such wonderful speeches.

After all the speeches were given, we each got our gifts and everyone had a nice talk with each another. It was October and we were then in Spring. So the warm, humid day ended with a thunderstorm. As the venue of the event was by the bay we were caught in the brunt of the storm as we were going home, yet we made it back safe and happy.

My final speech of that month was at a church up in North Lakes. This was on the evening of Sunday, October the 27th, which was two days before our departure to the US that year. North Lakes Anglican Church was hosting a fundraising event for autism, as this condition affects so many people and families within the community. There were three speakers including myself, my mother and a therapist from Brisbane. As well as speeches, there were also a large number of local organisations with stalls outside in the foyer; promoting the wonderful work they do for those of us with autism (or affected by the condition in other ways). That night ended up being a very enjoyable event for both me and my mum.

Two days later on Monday, October the 29th we left home early in the morning fully prepared for an exciting family holiday. Once we got to the airport we checked in our luggage straight away and then had breakfast. After breakfast I always like to look in the bookshop for something to during the long transit, and I bought a 3D jigsaw puzzle of a golden snitch from the *Harry Potter* series. The weather in Brisbane that morning was wet and miserable, yet I knew that we were soon going to fly above and away from that stormy weather.

Unfortunately our flight to Los Angeles was not a direct trip, so we had to stop off in Auckland for five hours on the way. We left Brisbane just after 10am and it took us three hours to get to Auckland. At the end of our New Zealand holiday three years beforehand, we enjoyed playing mini golf next to the airport in Auckland. Yet we weren't able to this time, as we couldn't pass border security.

In late October, New Zealand is three hours ahead of Brisbane. So it was evening by the time we completed this first leg of our trip.

I had a lot to eat on the plane and I wasn't hungry enough for dinner. Also, my body clock was three hours back in time. Our flight to Los Angeles wasn't until nearly midnight, and it was delayed for roughly another hour due to there being a thunderstorm.

Though I whiled away most of the time by doing mindfulness colouring on my iPad, as well as playing *Disney Magic Kingdoms* (which is a game from the App Store where you can build and manage your own Disney Park). Luckily the tables we were sitting at had areas where we could recharge our phones and iPads.

Gradually the thunderstorm settled down to the point where it was considered safe enough to soon take off. Then it was time for us to go through border security and make our way to the departure lounge. Currently it's policy for everyone travelling to the US (who isn't a US citizen) to have a face to face interview on their last port before entering the country. They also had to do each of us separately. Mum and Brent explained to them that I had autism, and that Kylie and Dylan had Intellectual Impairment.

My own interview went very well and the officer was delightful with me. I had to explain why I was going to the US, whether I had gone previously and I had to explain all the details about why I went on all of those occasions. When he heard about the HSAM research tests at the lab, and the media story I had done over there, he smiled and said that he was very pleased to hear that.

Everyone else's interview went well too, and when there was a slight hiccup with Dylan having difficulties with understanding some of the questions, mum explained that he had been assessed as having an IQ of 60. After hearing those words there were no further difficulties with his interview, and it ended very nicely.

Finally we reached the departure lounge and were set for a very long trip. But once we reached the gate Mum was told that she had a random number on her boarding pass, and she was required to go all the way back to border security for another inspection!

At this point we were literally at the door of the plane so I began to panic. Yet my mother gave me a Valium tablet and assured me that it would be fine, as did the cabin crew. We waited for around 15 minutes (which wasn't too long) and I was assured by the crew that they would hold off the flight until Mum returned.

A short while afterward, Mum had a chance to tell me what had happened once we were all in our seats and had taken off. The inspection initially wasn't good as their sensors detected restricted drugs (Valium) on her hands. Though after Mum explained that it was prescribed Valium of which she had just given her daughter, (with a doctor's note) they were very apologetic. Whenever they discover that a potential situation is related to a medical issue (and is both legal and harmless), they are almost always very apologetic and kind afterwards.

That night there seemed to be thunderstorm activity within much of the South Pacific, and that made the first half of the trip quite bumpy. However I was tired enough to find this somewhat relaxing to sleep in. It reminded me very much of the sensation of being rocked to sleep; and it brought back comforting memories from my infancy, when that sensation always made me feel so safe and secure...

Luckily I did manage to get six hours of light sleep, even though I did wake a fair few times as a result of the sharper bumps and jolts. However there were a relatively small number of people in our cabin, so we all had empty seats around us to gain much more comfort.

What was brilliant about this flight compared to previous ones we'd had, was that falling asleep for six hours (made easier by our later departure) virtually cut the travelling time in half. By the time we were halfway to our destination the flight was smooth and we were able to be served breakfast.

After I had finished my cereal and orange juice, I did a *Harry Potter* movie marathon to while away the remaining time. By the end of the flight, I had reached *The Goblet of Fire*, which is the fourth film in the franchise. Thus it was easy for me to make the decision of doing a marathon of the last *Harry Potter* films (and *Fantastic Beasts and Where to Find Them*) for the journey home.

Once we had landed at the LAX I was very exhausted. Despite sleeping for six hours, it was very light and broken sleep. While we were going through border security, Brent and Dylan were asked to lift up the heavier suitcases so that the officers could inspect them. However the words of which they used in the sentence, as well as the speed at which they were given were quite difficult for Dylan to understand. The officers gave Dylan a very suspicious look and Brent explained that he had Intellectual Impairment.

From personal experience we've found that many assume that Intellectual Impairment just means that the person has a minor learning difficulty, but not to a level which affects their ability to live independently. Mum and Brent then said that he had been diagnosed with an IQ of 60 (an IQ of 100 is average) and that he also had autism. Once they heard that he had autism the situation was cleared. We've found too that autism seems to be more widely heard of than Intellectual Impairment, even though many don't understand much about what autism is.

On a happier note, the place we were staying at for the first third of this trip was in Anaheim next to Disneyland. During the car trip to our hotel I was feeling a mixture of excitement about another happy holiday ahead, and a need to have a nice long sleep before the next morning. Fortunately we were then in the evening, and it was around dinner time.

On that trip we stayed at The Majestic, which is made to be the castle of Princess Corinne. As it was late October, the place was fully decked out for Halloween. I was very happy to see some carved pumpkins decorated as characters from my favourite Disney Pixar film, *Coco*. We'd been fed a lot during the flight, so I didn't feel up to having dinner. Though I did enjoy (by wearing earmuffs) the beautiful fireworks display visible from Disneyland nearby.

After a good night's sleep I woke up bright and early, looking forward to day one of an exciting holiday. For breakfast I had waffles topped with strawberries and cream, and it was delicious. The US do far better waffles and brownies than what we have anywhere in Australia. Once we had all finished breakfast, everyone was super keen to take an early shuttle to the Disney Parks.

While we were going through security prior to entering Downtown Disney, one of my stress balls that I bought on my Maitland trip fell out of my bag. When it hit the floor it cracked but was still useable. I was initially quite upset. But my mother, as well as the man checking my bag said that the crack would remain a souvenir of this happy holiday.

Eventually, we had finished going through security and it was time for us to get our weeklong passes printed. After that we had a look around Downtown Disney before entering the Disneyland park. A few changes had happened in Downtown Disney since my previous visit. It was sad to see that Build a Bear had closed. Though the Lego Store was still open (which I liked just as much), along with the World of Disney store. Due to it being Halloween time, there were carved pumpkin displays just about everywhere.

For every one of my Disneyland trips I've gotten Mickey ears to keep as a souvenir. In 2011 I got Sorcerer's Apprentice ears, in 2014 I got Mickey Mouse (the character himself) ears, in 2016 I got Mad Hatter ears, and in 2018 I managed to find Jack Skellington ears in World of Disney. This was prior to us entering the actual park, and meant that every picture taken of me throughout the Disney leg of this trip included me wearing those ears.

In the Disneyland park that afternoon we spent most of our time at Mickey's Toontown because it had been a long time since Kylie and Dylan had visited there. So we took updated photos of all of us in Pluto's doghouse and sitting inside Mickey and Minnie's homes. In addition to Toontown we also spent a lot of time in Mainstreet visiting the shops, seeing the parade and we even did a couple of train rides around the entire park.

It was nearly midnight when we returned to our beds, and after such a stimulating day I only realised how tired I was when I fell asleep instantly. It's fortunate that my usual amount of sleep (which enables me to feel rested and fully wakeful) is a mere four or five hours when it is very deep.

The next morning however I was feeling sore in the stomach and I hoped very much that this wouldn't ruin my experience of Halloween (on October the 31st). Yet mum always has perfect ideas and suggested that I have porridge (oatmeal) for breakfast, as this would make me feel better. At first, I was a little skeptical about whether this would work. Though I took mum's advice and was surprised that it ended up being a complete success.

We briefly visited Tomorrowland first thing in the morning, but we spent most of Halloween in Disney California Adventure. Prior to lunchtime (even though we skipped lunch for an extra large dinner) we visited Radiator Springs, and Kylie and Dylan got to meet Lightning McQueen and Mater for the first time. Afterwards, they went on a ride which featured Mater singing hilarious tunes while they were spinning around in carts. I chose not to go on that ride because I feared that I would get unwell again, and I was determined to enjoy this Halloween experience without feeling sick. Brent, Kylie and Dylan are always able to do spinning rides again and again without ever feeling motion sickness.

After they had all had a few rides we bought some milkshakes at Flo's Cafe nearby. Mum and I suggested this, as we remembered how nice their milkshakes were on our 2014 trip. Despite it being October the weather was still very warm, especially while we were in the sun.

Once we had all had one or two milkshakes we headed over to the Mike and Sully to the Rescue attraction, which was another suggestion from mum and I. Then after we all had a few journeys through Monsters Incorporated, it was time for us to do some more shopping, and to have a chai latte at Starbucks.

Eventually, when it was dinner time we went to Smokejumpers Grill where I had an extra spicy burger. Yet I passed the waffle fries to my brother as I have always found them way too oily. Greasy food makes me feel sick. After dinner we watched an Electric Parade featuring most of the Pixar characters, which was a great way to wind down before going to bed.

We spent the next day at the Disneyland Park, and not the California Adventure Park (where we had spent our time the previous day). First we visited New Orleans Square to see *The Haunted Mansion*. On previous trips when I had been on the ride it was the standard version. Though as it was Halloween/Christmas time, on this visit I got to experience the *Nightmare Before Christmas* version. I absolutely love *The Nightmare Before Christmas* film and my favourite character is Jack Skellington, so I was very pleased that I got to see this. It was fantastic to see Jack and all of his friends, as well as being able to go through a kitchen smelling of gingerbread cookies.

Next we visited Adventureland and I went on the *Pirates of the Caribbean* ride for the first time. I had known of this attraction for quite some time but had never gotten round to going on the ride. This was mainly because most of my other Disneyland trips were rather brief. Yet I finally got to go on the ride during this holiday and I thoroughly enjoyed it; so much so that I had a few additional goes. I like the *Pirates of the Caribbean* films very much and it was fantastic to see all of the animatronic presentations whilst riding the waves.

This put us all in the mood to see more animatronics, so we then went to another attraction that we knew well, which was the enchanted Tiki Room. We had seen this show on all of our other visits, and we had certainly not grown bored of it. After that show we (Kylie, Dylan and I) climbed Tarzan's Treehouse, and then we all boarded Mark Twain's Riverboat. Prior to having a turkey leg each for lunch, we saw a Dia de los Muertos (Day of the Dead) display from the film *Coco*.

Once we had all finished our huge turkey legs, we went to Mainstreet to watch a parade. While we were there we also came across two families who were from Australia (and Brisbane) like ourselves. Prior to travelling so far away from home, I used to laugh when people would tell me stories about becoming excited, whenever they met fellow Australians overseas. Yet nowadays I do finally understand, and words cannot exactly describe that excitement! After the parade had ended I bought some Halloween cupcakes from a cafe, and had a chai latte at Starbucks. There I also took a picture of my decorated cupcakes before eating them.

There was something else that I bought at the park in 2018, which had personal significance for us. The classic Mickey Mouse episode *Steamboat Willie* had its world premiere on November the 18th, 1928. This was also the exact date and year when Brent's father, George was born. So I was sure to purchase and take home one of the caps which featured the well known (monochromatic) picture of Mickey, whistling at the helm of *Steamboat Willie*.

Then it was time for Dylan's favourite moment of the holiday. Galaxies Edge wasn't yet completed in 2018. However there were still a reasonable amount of Star Wars experiences available at Tomorrowland.

While we were in that section of the park, we first met Darth Vader and Chewbacca. Darth Vader looked at Dylan's BB8 ears on his hat and said (in his deep voice) that his allegiance disturbed him. He was very much in character! Yet Chewbacca (Chewie) was very sweet and gave us all a hug.

The following day was our last (whole) day at Disneyland for that trip. Before having one last go on our favourite rides we visited World of Disney. There I bought a plush toy of Simba for my young cousin who adored *The Lion King*. Additionally, I purchased a box of plastic figurines featuring all the *Moana* characters, for myself. *Moana* is my next favourite Pixar film after *Coco*. Then I went into another store to buy a porcelain teapot set of Mrs. Potts and Chip for my sister Jessica.

That evening Dylan built himself his own custom Lightsaber at Tomorrowland, and at the Lego Store I bought a Hogwarts Express/Platform Nine and Three Quarters set, for me to put together once I'd returned home.

We spent most of the next day at the hotel packing up our bags, for checking out and boarding the cruise ship for the next phase of our holiday. Unlike our October/November trip in 2011 the weather was still very warm, so we took advantage of that and had a nice long day in the hotel's pool and spa. Mum also called our cousin who had her birthday on November the 3rd so that we could all send along our greetings (even though the US is a day behind Australia).

Finally we had dinner in Mainstreet at Disneyland, and everyone had a final look at the shops there. When we were in Pandora I saw some nice Disney charms. I had already gathered a collection of charms representing special mementos on one bracelet. Though the charms I saw this time wouldn't fit on my previous one. So I used the opportunity to buy a limited edition Disney Parks Pandora bracelet to begin another collection of charms.

By midnight we were all very happy about how the first phase of our trip had been. It was rather sad to say goodbye to Disneyland for a while, but we were also very excited about phase two of our awesome holiday. While we were having a late night tea and coffee at Starbucks, there was a picture in front of me, where Wendy was flying off to begin an unknown adventure with Peter Pan. Perhaps I could relate that to what I myself was experiencing at that particular time as well…

CHAPTER TWENTY-NINE

It was bright and early when we checked out of the hotel and took an Uber to get to San Pedro. This port was huge, even bigger than the one in Sydney.

Customs is always a scary experience for me and this was no exception. There were so many people hurrying in different directions, and it was almost impossible for me to know who was talking to who. All I could do was follow my mother's lead and ask her for clarification, if ever I didn't understand something.

While I was walking through the body scanner the alarm didn't go off so I continued to follow mum. Also there were people behind me impatiently waiting to go through, and I had been trained to know that it's okay to continue walking if the alarm doesn't go off, and when no officers ask me to go back.

Yet by the time I'd caught up with mum, I just realised an officer was talking aggressively to me. Though I couldn't understand what she was saying because she was talking too quickly, and I had a sensory overload from all the chaos and noise. So I asked mum in front for clarification of what she was saying to me, as I was rather frightened because the officer could have been saying anything to me. Then the woman became even more aggressive and said more slowly "No, don't talk to her. Listen to me".

I then had a meltdown because I felt that if I couldn't ask mum to clarify things which I didn't understand, it was a completely helpless (and scary) situation for me. A few minutes later I realised that mum had ushered me from the officer and had me sat in a quiet corner. Mum then said that she explained to the woman that I had autism, and that she understood more so when I began to have a meltdown.

Usually in situations like this, people have understood that I have autism as soon as they hear my verbal speech. I have a speech difficulty when it comes to using tone, and therefore my voice is monotonous and rather unusual. Though it is harder for people to notice this when I'm overseas, because it often gets passed off as just being a part of my accent.

Eventually I calmed down and became excited again about my upcoming cruise, and getting to visit Mexico for the first time. I have been in love with the Mexican culture ever since I was six years old.

Prior to boarding the ship we had to have our bags and bodies scanned again, and the officer this time was the polar opposite to how the previous woman was to me. I'm scared of going through customs and security checks, but it's certain that not all of my experiences have been terrible.

Once we boarded the cruise ship all of the previous anxiety had left me, and I felt excited about a whole new holiday ahead. Unlike our cruise in 2015 we had cabins with a balcony. So I spent much of my afternoon relaxing outside, watching cargo being loaded to and from this huge port, and finally taking pictures and videos of us setting sail.

Early next morning we reached San Francisco, and the Golden Gate Bridge (as well as the Bay Bridge) was beautiful to see as the sun rose. We also had a good view of Alcatraz from the window of the restaurant where we had breakfast before disembarking for the day.

San Francisco looked absolutely beautiful. As we were in November, the leaves had red and gold hues, though the temperature was pleasantly warm that day. First we crossed the Golden Gate Bridge on a trolleybus and Brent took a video from the top. The bridge was so long that it took us over a whole minute to cross it.

Then we did some sightseeing before walking over to Fisherman's Wharf to do some shopping. Here we found a huge candy store which sold every flavour of JellyBelly, and therefore I stocked up on Tabasco beans, and all the other kinds of chilli ones.

We were just about to head back over to the ship when Kylie spotted a Build a Bear store. I had been looking forward to making a bear as a souvenir for this trip, and that was the main reason for why I was so sad when I discovered that the store in Downtown Disney had closed. However now it was known to me that I could make this planned bear after all.

The five of us entered the store (as we are all Build a Bear collectors) and had a good look around at the merchandise. Our local Build a Bear stores are around the same size as the one we visited in San Francisco. However the US always have a few things which we don't have in Australia (and vice versa too).

CHAPTER TWENTY-NINE

Prior to making my new bear, I bought it a *Moana* costume as well as a few scents that we didn't have at home (which included Sugar Sparkle, Pumpkin Spice, Mint and Popcorn). I ended up making a bear named Sally, after the main female character in *Nightmare Before Christmas*. The scent I put inside her was Pumpkin Spice, which is mainly available in the US around Halloween time, and never in the Australian stores I visit at home.

After leaving San Francisco, we were at sea the entire time throughout the following day. However on cruises there is just as much to do onboard as there is on shore visits. During the morning we went to the sales and I bought a nice scarf, and then we visited the shop selling jewellery so that I could look at some charms for my new Pandora bracelet. Out at sea I did find it quite chilly for the first time in a while, so my new scarf came in handy whenever I had to go outside.

The next day was when the ship docked at Monterey. However we chose to stay onboard. I spent most of my time in the spa (it was quite warm when we were by the shore) and we also went to a mindfulness colouring class. Mindfulness colouring is a very calming exercise for me. With pencil and paper I enjoy using the *Harry Potter* and *Fantastic Beasts* adult colouring books. As well, I mentioned in class about some colouring apps I use, including **Colorscape** which turns photos we take on our smart devices into colouring pages. The guys running the class thought that the app sounded absolutely amazing!

When we docked at San Diego the following morning (Thursday, November the 8th), it was an onshore excursion we had all been looking forward to. However, there was a small incident which happened at the start of the day, while disembarking the ship. Due to having slight claustrophobia, I am always scared to use elevators. This is because I have an intense fear that I will get stuck inside that small cage and nobody will be able to get me out. So I always take the stairs. Yet Mum and everyone else took the elevator, and she told me to wait for them in the foyer where the elevator doors were; on the level they were going down to. This was because she wanted everyone to stay together.

While I was in the foyer however, security staff asked me why I was standing there, and I told them that I was waiting for my family to meet me; as I had been instructed by my mother to do so. The man then said "Don't mess us around today ma'am, we're not in the mood for it". For a few seconds I didn't know what to say and then the man told me where to go. Yet I struggled to understand what he was saying, because he wasn't speaking in a way in which I could understand. Due to my autism I have cognitive difficulties with being able to comprehend language that isn't given to me in a particular way. This embarrasses me a lot as well.

Though it scared me to think that I was likely to get arrested by them if I didn't move, so I asked him if he could explain to me more clearly as to where I had to stand; as I genuinely didn't understand what he was saying and I was very frightened. He then asked me "Do we really have to give you every single word?"

Luckily, at that point mum and the others came to meet me, and the man said to the other staff members "It's all ok, it turns out she really was waiting for her mother". This incident made me feel so down about myself. Firstly we always feel indignant (or even frightened) if ever we get in trouble for something that we're not aware of. But the main thing that hurt me was that he was ridiculing me for not understanding simple things. Questions were raised inside me as to whether I was indeed an 'idiot', because that was how he made me feel. I also got reminded of how I couldn't travel alone (which I had to force myself to accept after the Maitland trip), and there was this officer ridiculing me because I was a grown adult who couldn't understand instructions which were supposed to be simple.

After disembarking the ship, we said goodbye to Brent, Kylie and Dylan who were going to have a look at the old Midway Navy vessel. Though at that moment, I felt very depressed about my life and about who I was as a person. However I cheered up when I saw a beautiful 19th century wooden house. Once I had discovered that it was a museum that we could visit, I was delighted and so was mum! Mum likes everything to do with history as well.

A sign outside said it was called the Whaley house and that it was reportedly haunted. The sign also informed us that the place had been featured on a few paranormal shows. When the curators at the door greeted us upon entering, they asked me about what brought us there that day. I then told them that the small building looked so beautiful, and that I was in the mood for a history tour.

The curators were very friendly and when they asked us if we were 'spooked' we shook our heads and said that we weren't at all. When I entered the building it didn't feel scary or sinister. Instead I absolutely loved how the furniture and decor were set up to look like a time capsule from the 19th century. My local historical village is set up like this too, and I love visiting there on a regular basis. Therefore, this house gave me a comforting feeling of being back at home.

Though interestingly while I was taking photos in every room I could visit in the Whaley house, I noticed an unexplained apparition in one of the pictures I took on my iPad. There was a framed picture on the wall, and reflected in the glass seemed to be a woman wearing a large feathered hat, as well as a Victorian coat with a black fur collar. After seeing this photo, the curators were delighted about how clear this apparition was, and asked me if I could please share that image on their social media pages. I promised them that I definitely would.

When we had returned to the ship, I posted a selection of photos on my Facebook page, including the one with the supposed ghost. I had not captioned or given any other information apart from visiting a historical house which I really liked. Though three quarters of my friends and family spotted the apparition immediately, as they said that the woman was so clear. Initially they even wondered if there were mannequins or actors dressed like that in the house, and were astounded when I told them that there weren't.

Whether or not a person believes in ghosts or spirits, it's scientifically known that time physically exists, and time runs at a different speed depending on other conditions (or where we are) in the universe. In other words, time is neither uniform nor equal, and the past and future do also physically exist. So, I personally see no reason for why 'ghosts' cannot exist; as it makes perfect sense that various moments of time can occasionally become tangled and knotted. Perhaps certain people, technology or conditions can enable us to see these 'glitches' or 'imperfections' that time occasionally displays.

Next day came our excursion to Ensenada in Mexico. This was the day I was looking forward to from the moment of booking the cruise. Once we disembarked the ship we took a tour bus to a marketplace, and a stately building where we were treated to a mariachi performance.

When I saw Ensenada I was extremely satisfied because it looked very much like my favourite Disney film *Coco*, especially at the time of year when we visited. At the marketplace I bought a sombrero with a polka dot fabric bow on it, which I felt could pass as a sunhat whilst wearing it at home. I also bought a handmade plush of the main character of the film *Coco*, Miguel. While I was at Disneyland for Halloween there were plushes of the characters from *Nightmare Before Christmas* (I bought a Jack Skellington with his dog Zero) but none from *Coco*. So I was very pleased to have actually gotten one in Mexico!

All too soon it was time to leave this awesome place of the globe and set sail towards the final leg of our holiday. Prior to docking in Los Angeles we had a whole day at sea. In the morning we all watched *Coco* together (it was Brent, Kylie and Dylan's first time), then we spent the bulk of the afternoon packing up our luggage for when it was time to disembark the ship. That would be first thing the following morning. Finally, after dinner we all had one last look at the shops.

After the cruise, the final third of our holiday was Universal Studios (where The Wizarding World of Harry Potter is) and shopping at Citadel. Citadel is a huge mall of outlets, and we always do some shopping there whenever we visit Southern California. It is a slightly larger version of Harbour Town on the Gold Coast, where I occasionally buy clothes and shoes locally.

First of all we checked into our rooms at the Millennium Biltmore. This is such a beautiful hotel to stay at whenever we're in Los Angeles. It was built roughly a century ago and filming has been done there for countless movies, television shows and more.

After settling into our rooms we went to Citadel to do some shopping, as well as to have an early dinner. Whenever I visit the Converse store I always buy several pairs of shoes there. Converse sneakers are so much more expensive in Australia, and on that trip I bought four pairs for the price of one pair back at home. In the US, I also have countless more designs to choose from.

Brent was disappointed that the DC outlet had closed. However when he visited the Converse store for the first time, he ended up saying that he actually preferred the design and variety of their shoes. Thus, he informed me that I had changed his initial preference, from showing him the range of Converse shoes available on that trip.

Next to Converse was the Adidas store, and that's where I got Brendan another jacket to replace the one I bought for him in 2014. My mother's favourite store is Guess, so she had a good shop there for bags and purses. Finally we visited the Disney store before heading over to the eatery to have dinner.

For dinner we all had Subway and I got a 6 inch sub with tuna, olives and every kind of chilli/hot sauce available. Before heading back to our table Dylan was ordering his sub, with Brent helping him. It's unfortunate that Dylan has a speech impairment, which often makes it hard for people to understand what he's saying. This is made even more difficult overseas, and when he kept giving his order (without being understood) he ended up being very frustrated and on the verge of tears. Brent helped with Dylan's order, yet he too has a slight speech difficulty due to his dyslexia. As a result of that they couldn't understand Brent either!

Seeing that Dylan was upset, I then explained about his situation as well as I could. I wasn't completely sure if they would understand me. Though as they couldn't understand Brent and Dylan, I felt that there was no other option but for me to try. Luckily, they did understand me when I spoke, and they were very apologetic. So at the very least it did end on a nice note, and everyone was still able to enjoy dinner that evening.

After finishing our shopping at Citadel we visited Hollywood Boulevard. The shops there were great too, and from Hot Topic I bought a mini Newt Scamander suitcase, as well as a (non-edible) chocolate frog from the *Harry Potter* franchise. Eventually it was getting very late and we needed a good night's sleep for Universal Studios the following day.

Universal Studios is always an exciting trip for me. We left bright and early, so we ended up having breakfast at The Three Broomsticks. There are two main reasons for why we always eat at this restaurant whilst in Universal Studios. Firstly, The Three Broomsticks is from *Harry Potter*, and secondly the food there is always great and very affordable.

When we visited Ollivanders, I *finally* bought Fred Weasley's wand (which they had sold out of on my 2016 trip), as well as the entire *Crimes of Grindelwald* set of character wands. We did of course spend the whole morning at The Wizarding World of Harry Potter, and it's always the place where I spend most of my holiday savings.

However it was eventually time to move on (for that day), and after buying a heap of Butterbeers, we watched the Animal Actors show whilst sipping them. That show had generally remained unchanged since our 2011 trip, when Brendan was called on to the stage. Yet even so, the extraordinary animals in the show have never ceased to amaze me. Then after Animal Actors we saw the new Dreamworks 4D movie.

By that time I was feeling a lot of stress from sensory overload. However my favourite Dreamworks character is Gingy from *Shrek*, and seeing his funny acts lightened my mood considerably. After a long day at Universal Studios we had dinner at The Three Broomsticks before returning to the hotel.

The following day was Brent, Kylie and Dylan's final day of that 2018 trip. Mum and I stayed a few extra days as we had been saving up for the trip longer, and it was originally just going to be the two of us going. So after a buffet breakfast at the hotel we returned to Universal Studios, with Kylie's interest of *Despicable Me* and The Minions being our priority for that day. Brent and Dylan had previously had their Star Wars moment at Disneyland, and I had my *Harry Potter* moment the day before.

First of all we went on The Minions simulator ride, and while we were queuing up Kylie was happily answering all of the *Despicable Me* questions that were being asked. After having a couple of rides we visited all of the shops in that section of the park. Therefore, it was then Kylie's turn to spend most of her savings.

In the afternoon Mum, Brent, Kylie and Dylan went to do the Studio

Tour. I didn't go that time because I didn't want to experience the sensation of heat on my skin, from the flame thrower. So while they were visiting that attraction, I returned to the *Harry Potter* section of the park, where I had a butterbeer and watched the performances on stage.

Prior to saying our goodbyes to Brent, Kylie and Dylan, we had dinner at The Three Broomsticks. Then we returned to the hotel for them to all pack their bags ready for their long flight back home. Once the car came to take them all to the airport, we hugged each other and wished the three of them safe travels.

Though, after saying goodbye to them all, it gave me an uneasy sensation of emptiness within. With further thought it makes sense why I felt this way, as more than half of us had left our large family group that night. But the feeling also had loneliness attached to it.

Then after experiencing that, there was another feeling which came to me a few hours later. As I was falling asleep I intended to remind myself that I had a few extra days of holiday fun. However I was forced to admit to myself that after being in another country for three weeks, there was a part of me which missed home as well. This validated that I will always visit California regularly throughout my life, yet I still don't feel like I could live there permanently, as much as I dream of it happening one day (while I'm at home in Brisbane). There truly is no place like home. So my dreams that night were about me being in my own bed, and that bed was such a long road away…

Even so, I did still manage to have a great time the next day. We began by having breakfast at The Three Broomsticks, and then we spent some more time having fun at the Universal Park. We had a good look at *The Simpsons* section and I bought a Lard Lads donut for lunch (a holiday treat only)! Back in 2016 I got a supersized Homer Simpson donut (with pink icing and multicoloured sprinkles). Two years later, a little more variety was added to the range, so I then tried a cookies and cream donut, with crushed Oreos and white icing. It was sweet but delicious. However I wasn't brave enough to look at (or even think about) the amount of calories it contained! But with all of the walking around that I was doing, I was confident in thinking that I probably burnt off about half of those calories anyway.

While we were at the table eating, Mum called Nana so that we could tell her all about our fun adventures. This was a great experience because we were speaking about the fun of traveling, and Nana shared some of her own experiences from traveling abroad. So everything flowed very nicely.

Though after lunch my sensory overload peaked again, and I was on the verge of having a meltdown. Mum can always tell (before I myself can) when a potential meltdown is on its way. This is because my actions will always show particular signs. Early warning signs include moments when I completely misunderstand words in conversation, unintentionally raise my voice volume, shake my hands, hit my head, rock back and forth, or repeatedly ask/answer one particular question over and over again.

So my mother decided that we should see the Dreamworks 4D movie again. More of the *Harry Potter* section of the park would perhaps have worsened the situation for me at that particular time. My psychotherapist rightfully said that both excitement and anxiety have equal potential to create excessive stress and meltdowns.

However the Dreamworks film was good, as the character Gingy raises my endorphins as much as Mr. Bean does. The moment when Gingy teased the pink haired troll, Poppy (from the Dreamworks *Trolls* films) about saying 'doody' instead of 'duty' was when the anxiety vanished from within me. Gingy is so cute and hilarious whenever he behaves like a cheeky little kid!

From there we went over to the backlot so that we could get some fresh air and more views of the Hollywood hills. Located there were two of the steepest escalators I had ever seen in my life. They were so steep that while we were on them (going down) the ground to which we were travelling seemed to angle up towards us. This reminded me a lot of a scene in *Harry Potter and the Philosopher's Stone*, where Harry is steeply diving towards the up-coming ground on his broomstick; only to eventually fall and catch the golden snitch with his mouth.

Halfway down the first escalator my mother began to get frightened because she has an intense fear of heights. Unfortunately we had to travel all the way down before we could climb onto another escalator to take us back up. Finally we got onto that next escalator and mum was still feeling very uncomfortable; yet she felt a little bit better that second time, because at least she didn't have to see the ground angling up towards her.

Later that evening we had dinner at The Three Broomsticks. While we were there we received news on Facebook that the other three had arrived home. However their journey back home was quite stressful. They told us that they had been downsized to a domestic sized plane, and that the flight was so rough that they could hardly ever use the bathroom throughout the long journey. For an instant I felt like I had that whole experience ahead of me. It was difficult to work out whether Mum and I really were the lucky ones still on holiday, or if the other three were the lucky ones having now completed that long and stressful trip.

Yet those tense feelings soon lightened considerably, when we found out that there were tickets available to see a screening of *Crimes of Grindelwald*, in the IMAX theatre at Universal Studios. That was to be on the morning prior to our late night flight back home. This would work out well, as it would be a great way of winding down before having to make our way to the airport.

There were still two full days of our holiday before then however. The next day Mum and I visited Santa Monica peer which was an absolutely fabulous experience. Before going to the peer itself we had a walk around the shops and cafes, and at Starbucks I had a spicy chai latte. As well, I bought a bottle of water for while I was walking.

Eventually when we were on the pier (at the end of the world famous Route 66) the sea breeze was lovely, and so was the sight and sound of everyone having a happy time. Mum told me that she received memories from her early childhood, when she would occasionally visit Blackpool Pier in England.

While we were there filming was being done. But at the same time the pier wasn't closed, and there was a sign notifying guests that there would be a possibility of them being included in the film (if they were present in a certain area).

As always, whenever people are faced with this possibility there are half who feel excited about being on film, then there are others who shy away from the experience.

Returning to our hotel was a slight challenge due to heavy traffic. At that time the major highway from our home in southern Queensland was having major upgrades, and everybody was complaining about how much of a nuisance the traffic was. However when I was in the much more heavily populated city of Los Angeles that evening, I got to experience *their* version of heavy traffic. A trip which under normal circumstances would have taken around half an hour took nearly three hours instead! But on the bright side we had a chance to see (whilst in the car) many other nice places in Los Angeles that we could visit on our next California trip.

Once we had arrived back in downtown LA, we had another walk around the block to stretch our legs. Again we visited Starbucks (where I got a strawberries and cream frappe that time) and for dinner we went to a nice Singaporean restaurant attached to the Biltmore. I was pleased to be able to order super hot food there, which was spicy enough for me to like, even though I can have spicier meals. At the vast majority of places local to me (including Nandos), I will order extra-extra hot and it merely tastes like pepper.

The next day mainly involved us packing up our bags and luggage, so that we would be ready for our flight home the following night. That would also enable us to enjoy watching *Crimes of Grindelwald* without feeling rushed and stressed.

On the morning of our final day of the trip, we woke up early and triple checked that every possession was organised and packed. This was despite the fact that we weren't checking out until the evening. Prior to going into the cinema, I spent the last few dollars of my savings on candy to eat during the movie, as well as something to munch on during the long flight back home.

I was so pleased to see *Crimes of Grindelwald* at Universal Studios on the massive IMAX screen. Even though I would have seen the film a day earlier in Australia, it just wouldn't have been the same. We do have IMAX theatres in select places, but certainly not at my local shopping centre (where I would have otherwise seen the film). Waiting an extra day is definitely worth it and I was having weeks of fun on my holiday beforehand anyhow.

Sadly the evening came up quickly, and it was finally time for us to head to the airport. At that stage I was longing to be back in my own familiar environment, even though I knew that I would no longer feel that way in a few months time. Also, I really wasn't looking forward to the long, tiring flight ahead of me. I sincerely hoped that we wouldn't end up having the same experience as Brent, Kylie and Dylan did.

But, lo and behold, when we were waiting in the boarding lounge at 11:30pm we were informed of the very thing I was dreading. Our flight had been downsized to a smaller domestic plane. We were also told the same story (five days later) that the other three were given. Apparently the wing on the larger plane had received damage from heavy turbulence and for that reason they had to use a domestic sized aircraft. There were only three possible explanations for this story. The first was that they were lying, the second was that they only had one international sized plane, and the third was that their aircraft were of that poor quality they broke on every single trip.

From knowing that the other three were told the same story five days ago, my mother and I knew the truth. They had realised that a relatively small number of people were going to be on the plane, so they downsized the aircraft for the purpose of *them* saving money. However after acting out on this decision, there were too many passengers for one small plane, so we had to be split into seperate groups.

As soon as we began to taxi towards the runway the air conditioning was cranked right up to a very uncomfortable level. From take-off to the time we landed 14 hours later, the turbulence wasn't the worst that I've ever experienced. Yet it was enough that the one bathroom was closed to everyone for 80% of the flight duration. It was so bumpy that even the cabin crew had to be seated for most of the time. Being squashed like sardines for 14 hours, whilst being constantly rocked from side to side isn't at all comfortable.

Nobody slept on that flight, and the man sitting in front of my mother had his seat reclined into her chest for the full duration of the trip. He also ignored the flight attendants when they asked him kindly to straighten his seat, when mum was served a drink and meal. A woman we were speaking to said that she was a travelling nurse and flying was a regular part of her life. She told us that this was definitely the worst flight that she'd ever been on.

Over that 14 hour stretch of time, there wasn't a person onboard who seemed to be happy. As usual, it all ends with the words "I hope you enjoyed your flight with us" before the passengers disembark. However after this flight there were a few shouts from different cabins saying that it was a horrible experience and that they demanded a refund. Those who purchased business class seats were absolutely furious.

Also, once we had disembarked the aircraft, the abrupt response to mum's question of which gate we had to go to (for the next flight) was, "just walk into the building and find your way".

As this was Auckland, and not Brisbane, we had another three hour flight before we would finally be back at home. Prior to catching our connecting flight, border security gave my mother a random check, though once she had finished the officer was absolutely lovely to us. In fact, she was of so much more help than the cabin crew were.

It was a very tight connection between flights, and from that built up stress (as well as fatigue) I was beginning to have a meltdown. But we were kindly assured by the airport staff, that they would make sure that the plane wouldn't take off without us.

Unlike the longer flight, the one from Auckland to Brisbane was much nicer and smoother. Ironically we were in a larger aircraft for this short journey than we were for the previous one. I was very tired, but I knew that I couldn't have a nap when I was back home. We landed in Brisbane when it was the late morning and Brent had come to drive us home. On the way we were caught in traffic due to major roadworks on the highway. However at that time we just laughed, and felt like it was nothing at all!

After a week I had more or less adjusted to being back home, and in our own time zone. On Wednesday, November the 28th I had a travel training day with a support person, and I chose to go to Dreamworld. Our local theme park is minuscule in comparison to Disneyland. The whole park is slightly smaller in size than Universal Studios in

Hollywood. But I was super keen to get some more bricks for my Lego village, and to see the worlds of the Dreamworks films. At Dreamworld there is a section dedicated to the films *Madagascar, Shrek, Trolls* and *Kung Fu Panda*. While I was in the Dreamworks store I bought a plush Gingy holding a lollipop, which was exclusively made at Dreamworld. Also, like Disneyland and Universal Studios they offered meet and greets with a few characters.

I was delighted to find out that they offered a meet and greet with Gingy! At Universal Studios I kept saying to mum that after all the characters we met at Disneyland, I would have liked to keep a photo of me with Gingy. Unfortunately that didn't happen during the trip, because there wasn't a Gingy to meet and greet at Universal Studios. Though I was very pleased to finally have a photo with my favourite Dreamworks character a few weeks after then, at Dreamworld!

December 2018 marked the end of a year like no other, as it was jam packed with so much activity. That could easily have made the following year seem very quiet and boring in comparison. However, a quieter year would enable my mind to be less distracted, when it came to learning new skills and life lessons.

CHAPTER THIRTY

COMING TO TERMS WITH THE REALITY OF LIFE

Two weeks later on Tuesday, December the 11th it was my 29th birthday, which as always was a very enjoyable day. Then, on the following day I stretched out the fun by updating my Optus contract. I was finally ready to get my 256G iPad Pro 2.

As a Christmas and birthday month special I even got 100Gb of data free for each month of the two year contract.

This meant that after I paid for the general cost of my new iPad, I additionally had 100Gb of free data a month for two whole years! This was fantastic news as it eliminated my fears of having to do a media talk or presentation via video link, when our wifi was down at home.

On Sunday, December the 23rd we collected both Brent's mother and mum's mother and brought them to our house for Christmas. All of us being together was a tense experience at times. Though, I grounded myself by spending much of Christmas Eve re-painting one of the archways of my train set (which was being converted into a Lego Village). My intention was to make it look less like a tacky child's effort, and more like a realistic stone entrance to Hogwarts.

Christmas Day was spent at home where we talked, had our usual Christmas lunch, and eventually had dinner with three other family members celebrating alongside us. While Jessica was at home with us she mentioned to me that Stan (an Australian streaming platform) then had all of the Disney films and episodes of *Wizards of Waverly Place* available to watch. So I spent much of the next few days watching them.

After a whirlwind of a year in 2018, the following year may at first glance seem rather boring in comparison. But this certainly wasn't the case. It's true that I didn't have all of the travels and holidays. Yet those things are not what make a year exciting and productive. In many ways 2019 was a year when I started to (further) set my foundations for the future, and to begin taking all of the work I had previously done to the next level.

On Mum's birthday (Tuesday, January the 8th) I had an ABC radio interview. Mum herself took me along to the studio that morning and she said that it was one of her happiest birthday experiences, as the interview ended up going superbly. This made me feel very good.

Some other very significant and pleasurable experiences happened in the first part of that year as well. At the time, the day of the week when I would go out to do leisurely things of my choice (with a support person) was Wednesday. Yet it was decided that I should also go out at nighttime on another day of the week, and immediately there was a place that both my mother and I already had in mind.

Just prior to going away on our 2018 family trip, Brendan and I went to a *What's Your Superpower* sensory disco. *What's your Superpower* was a group for autistic children and adults, founded by a few people in the community of whom I am well connected with.

Activities provided at *What's Your Superpower* included a variety of things commonly liked by autistic people, such as jigsaws, chess, jenga, snooker, playing the musical keyboard and more. It was decided by my mother and I that on Friday nights (when the sessions were held), it would be a good idea for me to attend their meetings.

While I was there I mainly talked with others who had autism, as well as parents of autistic children. I also did jigsaw puzzles, which I have enjoyed putting together since my infancy. After a few months of me attending, *What's Your Superpower* became an online only group. Though I stayed in routine with my Friday night excursions by going out to dinner at Indonesian, Pakistani and Turkish restaurants. Also, I've continued to keep up with talk and news from *What's Your Superpower* via Facebook.

However on a vastly different and unrelated note, in March of that year there was a moment when I felt particularly down and depressed. At that time I was really being affected and hurt whenever I was told "you need to get a day job" and "you need to get a 'proper' career which doesn't involve you merely talking about autism".

When I had established my career as a speaker and writer, I felt a strong sense of accomplishment. Earlier in this book I've spoken about the days when I was a teenager (in the process of leaving school), and feeling very upset about how my future didn't look very promising. This wasn't in terms of earning money. The main concern was of me never finding my passion, and therefore never gaining emotional fulfilment in my life.

Looking back now, I already found emotional fulfilment by making a choice at fifteen that I was not going to give up on becoming the best person I can possibly be.

That positive feeling within doesn't come from being given money, and nor from earning it. It also doesn't come from actually *being* the best person in the world. In truth, it comes from us knowing deep within that we've become the best person that we *ourselves* can possibly be.

However in this phase of depression, I felt hurt and sensitive about people telling me "you should be doing and achieving more in your life". After writing the previous paragraph, it makes perfect sense to me as to why I felt so down whenever I would hear and/or relive those words. The truth is that it means so much to me, that it's crucially important to try my absolute hardest to become the best person I can possibly be.

So if I have a person saying that I'm not doing enough, I will then feel like a failure, because in my mind it must mean that my efforts are not working. But then again, I'm gradually beginning to learn that when it comes to myself, I must listen to my *own* beliefs, as nobody else knows who I am as much as I do.

The same goes for every other person as well, which gave me an idea. A positive idea which lifted away the depression I felt. I expressed to my therapist that I would like to begin an organisation that would provide programs, which would enable autistic people to discover where their true passion is, and to then find out how they want to personally use that in their life. I also wanted this organisation to cater for people on all levels of the autism spectrum, and to tailor each participant's program to their individual passions, goals and abilities. Also, the participants' goals about how to use their discovered passion in their lifetime doesn't solely have to be for career or educational purposes. It could also be purely for their psychological, social or emotional wellbeing.

Prior to expressing those plans, I did have this idea in mind for almost ten years. However I was previously much more limited due to things like NDIS funding not being present, me not being connected to as many people and networks, as well as me not being emotionally and cognitively ready to actually do such a thing. Yet after expressing my goals to my therapist at that time (in March of 2019), she felt I was then at the stage where I'd be able to officially start planning out my business idea. More of this was set to unfold throughout the second half of 2019, and into the beginning of the following year.

However, on the final day of April, 2019 I had a radio talk for a 3AW morning radio show in Melbourne, which I gave via a cross studio broadcast from the 4BC studio in Brisbane. So once again (by coincidence for the fourth year in a row), there was a media talk that I did on April the 30th!

This interview was around an hour long and the lead researcher studying my memory (at The University of Queensland) was also invited to talk alongside me on the show. Interviews for scientific episodes go for a little longer than commercial radio talks, and I was very happy about how well it went.

Additionally, (exactly) three weeks later we received some more positive news. One of the television shows that our family watch, *The Project,* contacted me via email, inviting my mother and I to appear on their show. Of course our immediate response was "yes"! The filming for that ended up being on Monday, June the 17th.

But simultaneously in June 2019, more filming for another event (our family film *Because We Have Each Other*) occurred. On the first day of that month I was filmed underwater in a family friend's swimming pool. June is the beginning of winter for us, and even in Brisbane (despite the days warming up pleasantly) the early mornings do still get very cold! However eventually it got to a stage when it felt much warmer to be in the water than outside in the cold air! That's when we were able to successfully film some footage of me recreating a womb memory. Yet once I stepped out of the pool, I was physically unable to stop my teeth from chattering!

The next day I was filmed at a local rollerskating rink **Digi Skate**, where the producers wanted to get some footage of me gliding through artificial fog. As the smoke machine used a substance which was friendly to people with skin allergies, I didn't get any rashes afterward. Also the effect of the coloured lights reflecting off the smoke, as I passed through it, was spectacular. Over the years there was a lot of footage taken for our film, and even those moments which didn't make it into the final product (merely due to the film having to be a certain length) have still been archived and certainly not discarded. Later on that evening our family were treated to Baskin Robbins ice cream.

Then (as mentioned earlier) on Monday, June the 17th, *The Project* came to our house to film the episode featuring my story. This aired on Friday, June the 24th with amazing success. The moment Waleed (who interviewed me) stepped through the door we recognised him immediately from the show. It was a delightful experience, as Waleed and the rest of the crew present that day were wonderful to both Mum and I.

As we moved into July and deeper into Winter, it became colder. On the first weekend of that month, Brent had a race in Warwick and on Sunday, July the 7th I went out with the rest of the family to watch him. Further inland it gets even colder (during winter), and out in places like Stanthorpe and Warwick it can even snow on occasion.

We left home before 5am and we were all rugged up in jumpers and beanies. The fog was very thick that morning. It was extremely difficult to see through, yet luckily there weren't many cars on the road. It was a two and a half hour drive and the sun rose along the way. Gradually we saw the bright rays appearing over the mountains, which were covered by mist in the countryside. The sight was absolutely beautiful.

Once we arrived at Morgan Park Raceway, our gazebo was already erected from the previous day (I myself didn't go out there on the Saturday). Breakfast was being served, though I had eaten before I left home and didn't feel too hungry.

Yet I enjoyed myself for much of the day by playing with my Rubik's Cube and watching all of the races that Brent participated in. We also sponsor the Turner brothers and we enjoyed watching every race they participated in. By lunch time I bought a steak pie and it was delicious (which surprised me somewhat as I don't usually like beef). Then Brent's brother Mark came along to give him some further support.

When it was just past 4pm we began to pack up our gazebo, trailer and belongings for our return home. I felt that the day was very pleasant. The sun was out that day, so it wasn't quite as cold as we had expected. One great thing about a sunny winter day is that sitting out in the sun (safely protected) makes us feel much warmer.

Once we were halfway home we stopped by a small restaurant for a rest, and for some dinner as well. I myself had some pumpkin soup with toast to dip into it, along with an energy drink.

August of 2019 was another eventful month for me. On Saturday the 10th I decided to give my bedroom a facelift with new furniture, to replace those which were looking very shabby after more than a decade. The previous night Brent had gone out to IKEA to buy (from my own bank account) a new daybed, desk, shelving unit, desk chair and bedside cabinet. Thus when I came home from Baskin Robbins, I had a somewhat large job of removing all of my possessions from my bedroom, and temporarily placing them into the living room.

Then I went to the spare room (where I ended up sleeping that night) while Brent began to dissemble all of my old furniture, and to assemble the new furniture. It was a very big job which took almost the entire Sunday. Though at 11:45pm I was finally able to sleep in my new bed.

The next day, I spent the whole of Monday sorting out all of my possessions, and placing them into their new positions in my bedroom. It was a long and tedious task because I own a lot of things! However I thanked my past self immensely for sorting through and discarding certain things (which were either broken or not used for a long time) during the previous Summer. Those past activities literally made this job a hundred times easier for me.

The following month Brent had his 50th birthday, and Dylan

turned 18. On Dylan's birthday (Wednesday, September the 18th) another story featuring my HSAM was published. This time it was in **Mamamia**. As usual I received many supportive comments, as well as some negative ones. There was one where a woman tagged my name in a Facebook comment (so that it would come up in my notifications), and gave a series of Pinocchio emojis to poke fun at my story. Due to my name being tagged in this comment, my friends and family on Facebook saw it too. Yet they assured me that it was unfortunately inevitable that there would always be some people who disagreed with any kind of story. I truly do believe and accept that.

However, this still wasn't the best news to hear as I was heading out to Guzman y Gomez with the family to have a celebratory dinner for Dylan's birthday. Though once I was eating a nice burrito, where they put extra hot sauce on just for me, I felt much better. All that mattered was that I had nothing to worry about, because I had done everything within the law by telling media the truth (and I signed a contract promising to do just that). But even so, after initially feeling upset, my thoughts and life eventually moved on as further weeks went by.

It was then almost a whole year since I had left for my 2018 holiday, and I had nostalgic feelings about what I experienced on that trip. This included *Harry Potter* world at Universal Studios. So I decided that it was time for another trip up to Samford where I could visit The Store of Requirement, which ended up being on Saturday, September the 28th. Quite some time had passed since I'd previously visited, and therefore plenty of new stock was available. Hence the reason why I always like to go there when there are several months between visits!

Some of the things I bought were the wand of Oliver Wood, two new *Harry Potter* themed bedspreads, and some edibles (including a chocolate frog and a Sorting Hat cupcake). The colour of the icing inside the cupcake reveals a Hogwarts house, and when I had bitten into the cake it contained red icing for Gryffindor. Despite my Hogwarts house being Ravenclaw, I was still in the mood to pay my respects to Gryffindor on that day.

The following month (October) of 2019 contained a few very enjoyable events for me. On Wednesday, October the 9th I attended my first Spanish class at the **Lapont Language Centre**. Lapont is a school in Brisbane which teaches people how to speak a variety languages. For each language there are five different course levels, where each are paid for individually.

The primary intention of these courses is to teach people how to not only know the language, but to also be able to speak the language in daily conversations. So rather than simply learning a heap of new words and phrases every week, we go straight into asking each other general questions by solely using the language, and answering in complete sentences. As a result of that many are often amazed about how far students have come by the time they have completed just the first ten week course. Then, by the time students reach Level 5 they're not to use any English whatsoever in class (for a duration of a few hours). It's an excellent way to both practice and learn!

After I reached the end of my first course, I discovered something quite interesting. Learning a new language isn't nearly as difficult as it seems. Even when we listen to ourselves while we are speaking in our mother tongue, we are in truth merely speaking in organised sentences (with set word structures) virtually all the time! We only have to slot in an adjective, adverb and noun here and there in order to create different sentences.

So while learning Spanish (for example) all we need to do is learn sentence structures, use them in appropriate situations, and quickly look up any words we're unsure of. Eventually we'll remember those words too, in the exact same way as we do with the sentence structures. In Spanish, verbs have to be conjugated depending upon the subject, as well as nouns and adjectives having to agree in gender. However with these conjugations they all generally follow a set pattern.

In addition to beginning my language classes, I did some other exciting things during the rest of 2019. On Monday, October the 28th I decided to go to **Australia Zoo** for the first time in my life. I'd wanted to visit the Irwins' home for a long time, and my new support person (Paul) suggested that we should visit that Monday.

Luckily the upgrades for the Gateway Motorway had finally been completed, and our drive up to the suburb of Beerwah (where the zoo is located on the Sunshine Coast) was only an hour! Once we arrived at Australia Zoo I was in awe of how fabulous it was. We first went to the Crocoseum to watch some shows relating to Australian wildlife and environmental conservation. Then I had a savoury pie for lunch, and we spent the rest of the afternoon walking through various worlds. These themed sections of the zoo included Bindi's Treehouse, Southeast Asia, Africa, Bindi's Island, and more. It was a fabulous day and after that experience I decided that I would definitely visit Australia Zoo again.

The following month of 2019 (November) was just as eventful and exciting for me as October was.

On Friday, November the 1st Dylan had his school formal, and he was the final child in our family to graduate. Parents and siblings were welcome to join this event and it was held at **The Calamvale Hotel**. We stayed there and enjoyed the celebration until it was past 11pm. Then straight afterward, the film crew for our family movie took us to the Gardens Restaurant at the **Greenbank RSL**, for a little discussion about the film's progress to that date. We were informed of some very exciting things, yet unfortunately I'm unable to speak about them here, because they're still confidential.

A week later, I had another exciting event of November 2019, that was just as worthy of looking forward to. On Friday, November the 8th I visited **Supanova** in Brisbane city. Unlike my previous two visits to this convention, I did not wear my Hogwarts robes. It was far too warm. Instead I wore the **BlackMilk** Quidditch shirt I bought on my 2015 visit to Supanova. BlackMilk is an Australian clothing brand which makes a variety of *Harry Potter* merchandise to wear, as well as that of other pop culture topics.

At Supanova 2019 I purchased the new Ravenclaw BlackMilk shirt, some limited edition PopVinyls to give as birthday and Christmas gifts, and even a *Harry Potter* (mini) PopVinyl advent calendar for myself.

Every part of Supanova is exciting, but there is one part of which I like the most, and that has always been when I've met actors who were in the *Harry Potter* and *Fantastic Beasts* films. In 2012 I met James and Oliver Phelps, in 2015 I met Matthew Lewis and in 2019 I met Alison Sudol (who plays as Queenie in *Fantastic Beasts*). At the event I got both a photo and an autograph. I also brought along my own version of Queenie's wand.

Meeting Alison Sudol was absolutely wonderful, and she truly is such a sweet and lovely person. While I was having my picture taken she even did an act with the wand I brought along. Afterwards Alison did a Q&A session and she didn't solely talk about her experience of playing the part of Queenie in *Fantastic Beasts*. She also spoke about the anxiety she experiences. When she was sharing this with those of us in the audience, I was very interested and attentive 100% of the time. This is because I could relate with what she was saying very well.

November eventually moved along, and the following month was when me and the rest of my family were preparing for my 30th birthday. That officially marked the first three decades of my life, and concludes my written story (within this initial book) that you have just finished reading.

Wednesday, December the 11th, 2019 was the day when I finally turned thirty, and the event was an absolute blast. The film crew were even up here from Melbourne to share the experience. Amazingly we still managed to do the traditional 'present an hour' procedure with all of the activity!

When I woke up in the morning I did an audio interview, and opened all of the presents my siblings gave me. Then around lunchtime we went to Jessica's house, where more recordings were taken as we greeted each other. For lunch we dined at Montezuma's, and the food was delicious! In my opinion the meal I had that day tasted much more like authentic Mexican food, than those available at Guzman y Gomez and Taco Bell!

After lunch I was very full but we managed to get lots of filming done at home. Prior to doing the cake, mum and I played a game of chess outside where I won the game. That was fortunate because it was very important for me to be in a positive frame of mind that day.

As this was a milestone birthday my parents bought me a Baskin Robbins cookies and cream cake. For regular birthdays we have mock cream cakes from Woolworths. Yet there is one small problem with ice cream cakes on a summer day in Queensland, as they melt rather quickly due to a combination of the warm air and the lit candles. But luckily it only started to significantly melt once the song had finished!

Later that evening I also had the final Spanish lesson of my Level 1 course. For half of the session we were given a hypothetical map of a city, and our task was to practice giving and receiving directions. Then afterwards we had an end of term celebration. I myself brought along a pack of assorted Krispy Kreme donuts which we all enjoyed thoroughly; and of course the whole class wished me a "Feliz cumpleaños"!

It was then when I truly felt that a new chapter of my life had begun. I didn't have a firm understanding of this emotion. However the best way I can describe it is that I found myself thinking about the future.

As you have just read in this book, my lifetime memories from the past have repeatedly come back to me, both inwardly *and* outwardly. I'm constantly reliving distant memories, and I've now fully excepted this as a part of my life.

Yet, as has also been mentioned in this book, many external memories (such as people, events or even coincidences of calendar dates) also seem to reappear from time to time, as abruptly and unexpectedly as they disappear.

Personally, I'm currently uncertain as to whether these are purely and simply coincidental, or if the old phrase of "ghosts of the past will always continue to haunt us" is in fact true.

If that is indeed the case, then there are many more shocking surprises in store for me; some pleasant and others unpleasant.

There's no possible way that my own experiences in life would be any different from the kinds that other people experience. Yet perhaps it's easier for a person to see life's many coincidences, when they can remember every date and event that they've experienced.

Life truly is mysterious, and life truly is a puzzle for each individual to observe, work through and solve.

Acknowledgments

Thank you to Lynette, my life-long travel companion, for her generous encouragement and patient support during the writing of yet another book.

Thank you to my daughter, Naomi, to my good friends, Mark and Vivienne Moncrief, and to the leaders and people of E5 Elim Church Bristol, for their continued interest and enthusiasm.

My thanks also to Marko Joensuu (iheringius.com) whose diligence, creativity, and encouragement continues to be a source of inspiration to me.

Dedication

I dedicate this offering of worship to our Lord and coming King, Jesus Christ, the Alpha and Omega for all humanity, whose return will restore all things into a glorious consummation and wholehearted communion with God the Father. May our lives honour him and fulfil his purpose for us. To him be all the praise and glory, now and forever. Amen.

www.ingramcontent.com/pod-product-compliance
Lightning Source LLC
Chambersburg PA
CBHW050029090426
42735CB00021B/3421